# What Living as a Resident Can Teach Long-Term Care Staff

# What Living as a Resident Can Teach Long-Term Care Staff

## The Power of Empathy to Transform Care

by
Leslie Pedtke

Forewords by
William Keane, MS, MBA
Zoe Dearing, BME, MT

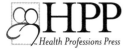

Baltimore • London • Sydney

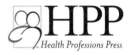

Health Professions Press, Inc.
Post Office Box 10624
Baltimore, Maryland 21285-0624

www.healthpropress.com

Interior and cover designs by Mindy Dunn.
Typeset by Absolute Service, Inc., Towson, Maryland.
Manufactured in the United States of America by Versa Press, East Peoria, Illinois.

The information provided in this book is in no way meant to substitute for a medical practitioner's advice or expert opinion. Readers should consult a legal or healthcare expert for further advice or information and for applicable regulations, policies, or practices in their own state or jurisdiction. This book is sold without warranties of any kind, express or implied, and the publisher and author disclaim any liability, loss, or damage caused by the contents of this book.

**Library of Congress Cataloging-in-Publication Data**

Names: Pedtke, Leslie, author.
Title: What living as a resident can teach long-term care staff : the power of empathy to transform care / by Leslie Pedtke ; forewords by Zoe Dearing, William Keane.
Description: Baltimore : Health Professions Press, Inc., [2017]
Identifiers: LCCN 2017031968 (print) | LCCN 2017031537 (ebook) | ISBN 9781938870477 (epub) | ISBN 9781938870453 (pbk.)
Subjects: | MESH: Long-Term Care—psychology | Attitude of Health Personnel | Health Personnel—education | Empathy | Caregivers—psychology | Quality of Life
Classification: LCC RT120.L64 (print) | LCC RT120.L64 (ebook) | NLM WX 162 | DDC 610.73/6—dc23
LC record available at https://lccn.loc.gov/2017031968

British Library Cataloguing-in-Publication data are available from the British Library.

# Contents

# About the Author

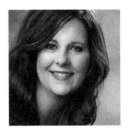

LESLIE PEDTKE, **LNHA**, is Educator for Quality Improvement for King Management Company. She worked as Administrator of Aviston Countryside Manor from 1994 until 2017. Through her experience of more than 20 years, she has built a foundation of person-directed care at Aviston as well as at King Management's other long-term care and assisted living communities.

During her time as administrator, Aviston Countryside Manor was featured in the 2013 spring/summer *LTC Today* ("Aviston Staff Walk in the Residents' Shoes"); the March 2012 issue of *McKnight's Long-Term Care News* ("You're Hired"); the spring 2011 *LTC Today* ("Consistent Assignments"); the April 2010 issue of *McKnight's Long-Term Care News* ("Empathy Crash Course"); and the Health Care Cost Insitute's (HCCI) Members Only newsletter for the intergenerational program Bringing Residents' Stories to Life. She was named one of HCCI's 2010 Heroes in Long-Term Care.

Leslie is currently Board President of the Illinois Pioneer Coalition, a Professional Educator for the Alzheimer's Association Greater Missouri Chapter, and a national presenter on the topics of learning empathy, best hiring practices, eliminating restraints, and decreasing falls. She is a graduate of Southern Illinois University at Carbondale with a B.A. in Speech Communication.

# Acknowledgments

I CONSIDER MYSELF TO BE A VERY LUCKY PERSON. My life has been touched by hundreds of people throughout the years who have taught me things I could never have learned in a classroom.

Often families tell us that they could never repay us for the kindness and care we have given to their loved ones. They do not realize that they already have thanked us. By giving us the opportunity just to be with their loved ones, to learn from them, is a gift. Thank you for sharing your loved ones with us. Bill, Larry, Beatsy, Dorothy, Les, Ruth, Evlyn—the list goes on and on . . . I will never forget any of you.

To the staff who moved into the nursing home, for the sacrifices you made for the sake of learning to be a better care partner, THANK YOU. The lessons learned from you have been invaluable to your colleagues. I am humbled by your perseverance, strong will, and integrity.

To Gary Glazner: By happenstance you were the catalyst who caused me to put this experience into words on paper—thank you.

To my mentor and friend, Zoe Dearing: You have taught me so much. Words cannot begin to describe how indebted I feel for the knowledge you have shared with me.

Finally, to my family: Thank you for your support and patience as I have grown and learned along the way. Without you, I may have quit after that federal survey and never looked back.

# Foreword

ALBERT EINSTEIN ONCE SAID THAT "there are only two ways to live your life. One is as though nothing is a miracle. The other is as though everything is a miracle." Leslie Pedtke's inspiring book is, in a sense, a bit of both in tracing the real-world journey of one nursing home administrator and her remarkable staff and how they learned about the power of empathy to effect meaningful and sustainable change in care and quality of life for residents.

My perspective on the subject of this book is both personal and professional. I have worked in the trenches of research and program development, promoting and supporting meaningful change and professional growth in long-term care as it revolves around the model broadly called "culture change" and its focus on person-centered care. Even well into the 21st century, there remains great resistance to this change model.

On the personal side, my mother lived through 12 years of advanced dementia in an institutionalized nursing home setting, where I visited her daily in the 1980s to ensure she was receiving some level of person-centered quality of care. Years later, a return trip to the nursing home revealed disappointingly few of the reforms and innovations that were making the rounds under the name of culture change. Other skilled nursing providers were only modestly better. For example, one nursing home administrator I met said he had mastered culture change by offering to residents the freedom to sleep in, engage in pet therapy, and enjoy buffet-style dining.

Although these may all be improvements in resident life, they remain somewhat superficial and not a fundamental change in the attitudes and practices within a community. Some other providers have focused instead on improving their listening skills and have recognized that, as you truly change a care community's culture, the staff, families, *and* residents will respond in meaningful ways. Leslie Pedtke is one such administrator.

Raised in a southern Illinois long-term care family business, Leslie launched into her own career as an administrator at one of the skilled nursing homes owned by her family, Aviston Countryside Manor. Her first federal survey, however, yielded more than 27 citations and dashed hopes for a successful career. After much research into culture change through organizations like the Illinois Culture Change Coalition, Leslie's solution—and revolution—began with a program she named Through the Looking Glass to help teach staff empathy.

To shift from a medical to social model of care, Leslie challenged her staff to voluntarily participate in a "contest" whereby they would move into the home and experience firsthand the challenges of living with the many effects of aging. The work focused less on paint and procedures—a common misdirection of culture change initiatives—and more on values and relationships. More than a dozen staff from various departments responded and lived as residents for as many as 10 days.

As you read through the staff's unique experiences, you learn about the challenges of loss; learned helplessness; the role of care partner vs. caregiver; the meaning of loneliness; the need to "slow down"; the effects of incontinence; the importance of communication; the meaning of "behaviors"; the role of family; and much more.

You will be fascinated by the lessons learned from the staff experiences of Through the Looking Glass, many of which have led to important, systemic changes at Aviston, including the elimination of personal body alarms and reduced falls. Aviston has also implemented a mandatory 24-hour resident "shadowing" experience for all job applicants, which has had a dramatic and positive impact on recruitment, training, and retention outcomes by helping staff to focus on *person first, diagnosis second*. Other effects included greater staff empowerment, the commitment to consistent assignments, and establishing a resident hiring committee with the power to make decisions—all examples of the risk-taking that is an essential element of culture change.

The true bottom line is that teamwork + research + a lot of risk-taking + a flexible blend of leadership can equal a lot of person-directed care. While still a work in progress, much of the success achieved by this rural for-profit skilled nursing provider in transforming its care practices is grounded in Leslie's willingness to give us an interactive peek through the looking glass of what it's like to live as a resident. I, for one, am thankful, and I urge you to put this book at the top of your "must read now!" pile.

Bless you, Leslie!

**William Keane, MS, MBA**
Consultant in Aging

# Foreword

I FIRST MET LESLIE PEDTKE IN 2007 when I went to Aviston Country-side Manor to talk to her staff about how to "deal with the behaviors" of people living with Alzheimer's disease. I remember that class very distinctly. As the Professional Education Coordinator for the Alzheimer's Association St. Louis Chapter, I was often called by different administrators or directors of nursing to come to the rescue of their staff who were struggling with trying to handle and understand the daily challenges in caring for people with memory loss. I knew that day that Leslie had something special in her approach to being an administrator. She sat quietly in the back corner of the room, intently listening to me and to her staff. When she spoke, she was bone honest about her own experiences and inquisitive with her thought-provoking questions. I could tell she *really* wanted to understand how person-directed care in its true definition could be relevant for people with memory loss.

Time and time again when I came to her community to educate her staff on various topics, Leslie took in information like a sponge, always taking something that she learned to create something even better from it and continue to improve on it. That is exactly what she has done with Through the Looking Glass, an inventive and inspirational program.

While we were having lunch at a local café one day, Leslie told me about this idea she had to teach empathy to her staff. Since then,

I have had the privilege to watch the seed of this creative thought turn into a beautiful and fruitful program that should become a model for the way we all orient our staff (and future staff) into the world of elders who are living in long-term care—most doing so not by their own choice, but because it is simply the cards of life they have been dealt—and who are so full of life.

I know many of the individuals who bravely offered not only to live as residents, but also to honestly reveal their feelings, good and bad, about their experience. I applaud them for the work they have done. I do not think they realize that they are also pioneers! I am mostly so proud of Leslie's leadership. She has become one of the "exceptional ones"—an administrator who other administrators would want to emulate.

This book is honest and candid—just like Leslie and her staff. There are no pretenses. This is exactly the way Through the Looking Glass put Aviston on a firm path to adopting person-directed care practices by having staff walk in the residents' shoes. Leslie's willingness to be open to finding a better way of care partnering and her humble vision of this program for everyone to experience is a great gift to her staff as well as to our elders and their families. She has changed the world of long-term care and made it a better place. In my nearly 40 years of working with people experiencing dementia and being a pioneer in the culture change journey, I have been given a rare gift, as well, to be part of Leslie's and her staff's journey.

I promise as you read this book that you will walk the journey with Leslie and her team and be inspired to embark on your own culture change walk into a better future for the elders in your care.

Go forward and make your imprint in the road.

**Zoe Dearing, BME, MT**
Professional Education Consultant
Board Member of Missouri's (MC5) Pioneer Network Coalition

# Preface

IN 1994, I BEGAN working as Administrator of Aviston Countryside Manor, a skilled nursing community in Aviston, Illinois. During the decade that followed, I had felt as though we were living survey to survey, doing our best to follow regulations while keeping our residents and employees happy at the same time.

On a hot and sunny day in August 2004, two women walked into our building and introduced themselves as surveyors from the Centers for Medicare and Medicaid Services (CMS). I stood motionless at our front door just staring at them. "We are from the federal government here to do a Federal Oversight Survey," one of them said. "I know," was all I could manage to say in response. As if it was not already hard enough having surveyors from the Illinois Department of Public Health (IDPH) do our annual survey, now we were having a Federal Oversight Survey (FOS)—a survey of our survey. The federal government surveyors wanted to make sure the state surveyors were doing their job. Our facility was bursting with anxiety and tension. There were tears, anger, and exhaustion among everyone involved. I experienced my very first panic attack.

The FOS ended as badly as it possibly could have. We received 27 citations, three of which were Immediate Jeopardy, meaning that a crisis situation existed in which the health and safety of the residents were at risk. One of the Immediate Jeopardy tags was

F490 Administration: *A facility must be administered in a manner that enables it to use its resources effectively and efficiently to attain or maintain the highest practicable physical, mental, and psychosocial well-being of each resident* (CMS State Operations Manual).

This was a tag about me.

Me.

Our residents were at immediate risk, and it was my fault. To be honest, I was doing a terrible job administrating, guiding, and leading this community. In fact, I was so bad that the Regional Director of IDPH made a personal visit to hand down my sentence following the FOS. I was to have a federal monitor check in on me weekly and another licensed nursing home administrator with me at all times to ensure I was not putting our residents in further danger. This went on until our facility was considered to be back in compliance, which was not until the day before Thanksgiving of that year.

By that time, however, I was done. Something had to change. I wanted out of long-term care. I saw the regulators and surveyors as the enemy, and the residents were suffering because of me. I began looking for a different job. Our community deserved someone who knew better and could do better.

But in the end, I could not leave. Long-term care was all I knew. I grew up in the business. My parents had owned and managed nursing homes since I was a baby, including Aviston. My father had been relentless in asking me to work for him. He expected me to want to be there. I felt guilty for wanting to turn my back on that. I stayed, but it took me a while, a year really, to pick myself up and brush myself off after that survey—and even longer before I was ready to hear that something good could actually come of the experience.

Then, in 2008, I learned of an organization called the Southwestern Illinois Pioneer Coalition and this new idea of culture change in long-term care. I listened hard because I had a feeling that this was what I had been looking for. It did not take long for me to be convinced that changing our culture of care was what we needed to bring joy back into our community. Let me be frank: If I was not happy with my job, how could any of our staff or even our residents be happy? Negativity is contagious. But so is being happy. I wanted to be happy where I worked—and I wanted our staff and residents to be happy as well.

Culture change became our revolution. We became soldiers of change, and everything we looked at, every practice we did, we wanted to change it. I began to realize during this revolution that change and transformation is also about building relationships, making connections, trusting each other, and being passionate about the goal. This was a lot more challenging. How could I get my staff to make that connection with the residents? I certainly cannot make people love their jobs and connect with those they are caring for. That commitment already has to be in their hearts. I just had to find a way to pull it out of them.

Culture change transformation is hard. Not everyone believes in it and many who want to really have no idea what it is supposed to look like or how to get there. Most of those working in our community wanted to get there, but we were not getting there fast enough and we did not know how to effectively approach culture change.

I chose Through the Looking Glass as the name for our effort to transform our care practices by teaching staff empathy. The program catapulted our community into creating an entirely different approach to how we care for the people who come to live with us. Whether a person moves in for short-term rehabilitation or long-term care, our approach became unified—*person first, diagnosis second*. We began marching to our own drum, and through our shared commitment we became unique in our community.

In this book, you will learn how we came up with the idea for our empathy program and the lessons our staff endured to become better caregivers and to teach each other new approaches to not only caring for those who live with us, but also caring with them. You will read journal entries from the staff participants that reveal powerful insights into what they learned. Every participant said the physical challenges, although uncomfortable, were not as difficult as what the experience of the program did for them emotionally. Each participant was stripped to the core before truly understanding what empathy is in caring with our residents.

In the months and years since the birth of Through the Looking Glass, relationships, connections, and passion have flourished beyond my expectations. A simple idea of asking staff to walk a mile in the shoes of a resident has gotten more attention than I ever expected. It is my dream that everyone working in long-term care takes the whole program or pieces of it to transform the culture of their community.

Amazing things will happen. Trust me.

The photos on the pages that follow show just some of the staff experiences of Through the Looking Glass.

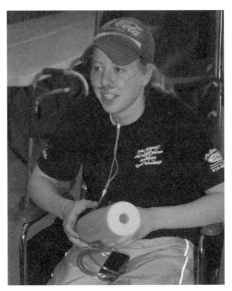

Nikki, certified nursing assistant, took part in a restorative program during her experience of Through the Looking Glass.

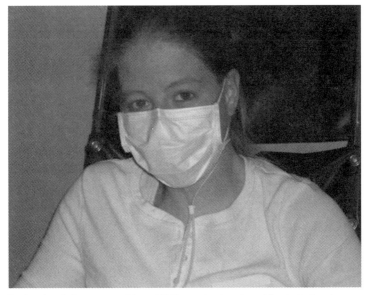

During her 6 days as a resident, Nikki was tired, sad, and frustrated and felt guilty for feeling tired, sad, and frustrated. The main lesson she learned through her experience was to slow down and take more time with the residents.

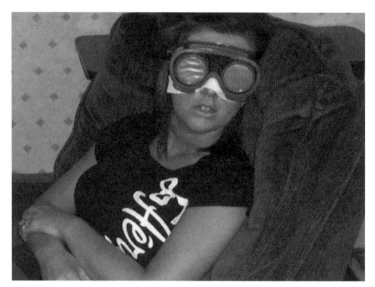

Amy, assistant director of nursing, spent the majority of her first day rocking back and forth in a chair. I later learned that the reason she stuck tissues in her vision-impaired goggles was because she could not stop crying.

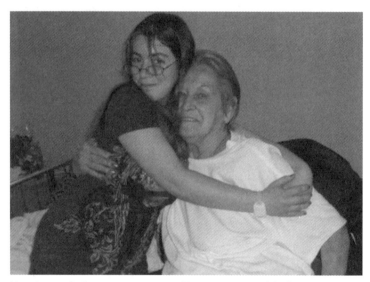

Victoria, certified nursing assistant, and her roommate, Mildred. During her 8-day stay, Victoria learned about the importance of talking to residents and asking them what they want (food, drink, activity, etc.).

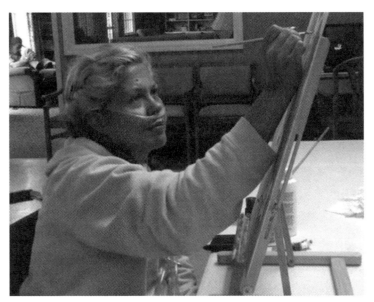

Jenny, who worked as a unit aide, found moments of joy in her day as part of her experience when she was able to do the things she loved.

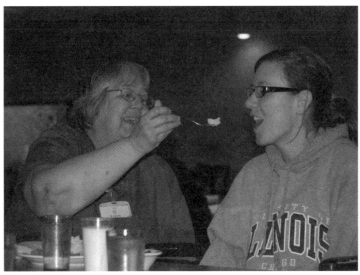

Karen, certified nursing assistant, feeds Lori, occupational therapist and participant in Through the Looking Glass. Lori had drawn the challenge that she had to be fed by a CNA who did not ask about her food preferences.

# Prologue
## Through the Looking Glass

As is standard practice in long-term care, we would conduct continuing education for staff with 30-minute meetings on paydays. We covered the required mandates as dictated to us through guidelines issued by the Centers for Medicare and Medicaid Services (CMS), and checked each off our monthly to-do list. When we identified a problem, either through our annual survey or from a resident or family complaint, we approached it in the same way, by offering staff in-services on the changes we needed to make. This approach rarely made a difference because, like many long-term care communities, we were experiencing high staff turnover. Change was almost never sustainable.

As an administrator, my primary job was dealing with complaints from staff, residents, and families—putting out fires before they became uncontrollable blazes. No one's voice was really being heard because we were too busy taking care of the "crisis of the day." Who had time to sit down and actually collaborate to find the root cause of a problem? The staff and I were too exhausted to investigate the "why" and were becoming more and more burned out.

When I first learned about culture change, it sounded like long-term care utopia to me—a world where everyone lived and worked together harmoniously. Was it too much to ask? Maybe. I just really wanted everyone to be happier. I wanted most of all for everyone, staff and residents, to want to be here in our community—living and working together. I became excited about the prospect of changes that could actually be sustainable.

Culture change is a transformation from the medical model (diagnosis guides the person's care) to a person-directed model in which residents and caregivers have a voice in practicing self-determination in their daily lives. Everyone is on a level playing field, with the needs of the residents leading the way.

In 2008, Aviston Countryside Manor, along with three other communities, had the opportunity to be part of a collaboration with the Southwestern Illinois Pioneer Coalition. The concept of culture change was still fairly new and the goal was to jump-start change through education and idea sharing. The experience was vital for our team. We began to take baby steps in changing our medical model into a person-directed care model. We painted bathrooms and bought pretty pictures depicting "home." We began using bread makers and making homemade soups. At the time, this is what we thought culture change was all about—changing our community into a more homelike environment for our residents.

That same year, I heard Carter Catlett-Williams, a founder of the Pioneer Network, say: "It doesn't matter how pretty you make your bathrooms if I'm not able to use them." This statement hit me like a ton of bricks. Our freshly painted bathrooms with pretty pictures on the walls and the cabinetry we used to hide sterile gloves and Depends did not really matter? We had been so proud of our accomplishments, which now seemed so trivial. Culture change transformation was so much more than changing the aesthetics of our building.

Additionally, our steps early on were not having an effect on staff turnover. We were spending so much money on help wanted ads that read *Come Join Our Team!,* with a picture of the director of nursing or certified nursing assistant standing next to a resident. We spent a lot of time trying to get the ads just right so people would apply, but spent no time thinking about what type of person we should be hiring and what our expectations of that person should be as part of a person-directed care model.

We needed *REAL* impact.

I continued to search for staff satisfaction that did not look like a pizza party or pay raises. And what about the residents? How could we teach the staff to improve their approach to care beyond an in-service of feeding each other puréed food or about having impaired vision?

Things began to change one day in the spring of 2009.

During a daily nursing report, I learned that one of our residents was dying. After I left report that morning, I wanted to say good-bye to her, so I knocked softly on her door and stepped inside. As she lay in her bed, I sat close to her, held her hand, and prayed. She did not open her eyes. I could not sense whether she even knew I was there. As I got up to leave her room, something inside me told me to stay. I closed her door and sat back down.

As I watched her and listened to her breathing, I wondered what it must be like to be her. She was dependent on us to take care of her, and now she was dying here in our nursing home. The silence of the room wrapped its arms around us. What was she thinking about? Her first love? The day she got married? Maybe she was thinking about the warmth of the sun and the sounds of the ocean, or the places she had visited or never had but always meant to.

I wondered if she was thinking about how she came to live here—and if she was afraid of dying alone.

As her life was ending on this side of the door, everyone else's was going on as usual outside of her room. There were excited congratulations to a certified nursing assistant who just became engaged, and another person was taking lunch orders for her co-workers. Everyday life continued.

Could she hear all of that? The world as she knew it was moving on without her. I wondered what that must be like. How did all of the residents feel, not just her, listening to all the activity around them and not being able to take part without asking for someone to help them? I was suddenly full of questions that I could not know the answers to unless I stepped into her shoes and lived on this side of the door with her.

Hmmm, I thought—now there is an idea.

After I left her room, I began putting some thoughts together. What if I asked the staff to move into the nursing home and live like the residents have to live? I could give them a diagnosis, such as congestive heart failure or a recent stroke, and they would have to role-play that diagnosis for the entire time they lived in the home. Every day they would be given additional challenges to deal with, such as being incontinent of urine, being bathed by staff, or losing a favorite outfit or pair of glasses— challenges our residents deal with all the time and that are a part of daily life in long-term care. Each day the challenges would be emotionally and physically harder on them. Like a game or a contest—who can survive the day-to-day of living in long-term care? More important, what could staff learn from participating? My hope was they would have a better understanding of the people they were caring for through the looking glass of experiencing the daily challenges they faced.

I was really excited and could not wait to share this idea with whoever would listen. I discussed it with other department team members, the Illinois Department of Public Health, our liability insurance company, and my family, who owned and managed Aviston. Not everyone thought the idea was a good one. Even my sister, whom I worked closely with, thought it was crazy and that no one would participate. I was not even sure myself.

After several months of mulling it over, I decided to introduce the idea to the rest of the staff. I placed a note in our break room announcing an all-staff meeting to discuss Through the Looking Glass. When the meeting time came, the room was packed with interested, curious staff. I was ecstatic!

I introduced the rules:

1. Contestants must replace themselves on their work schedule for the duration of the time spent as a resident in the nursing home.

2. Based on bed availability, it is preferred that ALL contestants participate at the same time.

3. Contestants may not leave the premises of Aviston Country-side Manor unless it is on an outing sponsored by the nursing home. If a contestant needs to leave, it must be approved by the Administrator and the time away will be deducted from the total time in residence.

4. Contestants must simulate a randomly drawn diagnosis when they move in. Refusing to participate fully may result in disqualification from the contest.

5. Contestants agree to daily "challenges" to simulate life in the nursing home.

6. Contestants agree to keep a journal of their experiences and are videotaped for the purpose of education and training.

7. Contestants agree to (1) create learning opportunities with their co-workers in their daily jobs and (2) participate in educational programs outside of our community with other organizations.

8. Contestants will be paid for the time they would have been regularly scheduled to work.

*Rules are subject to change at the discretion of the Administrator.*
*Grand prize of $500.00 for the person who stays the longest!*

I waited. Were they going to tell me I was crazy? I asked, "Who's interested?" Several people raised their hands.

I could not wait to get started!

PART ONE

# A Lesson in Empathy

# 1

—— • ◆ • ——

# Setting Goals to Change the Culture of Care

THE GOAL TO BEGIN Through the Looking Glass was multifaceted. We wanted to teach empathy and promote culture change in our long-term care community by looking at our common practices and asking ourselves, "What isn't working?" and "What would we like to see change?" We also looked at common complaints from the families of our residents as well as recurring citations from our annual state surveys. The practices we chose to tackle through the program were the ones that were having the most negative impact on our residents and that we were getting the most push-back on from staff.

I wanted our staff to feel what it is like not to be able to move without a personal body alarm going off, how painful it is to sit in a wheelchair for hours on end, or how it feels to be incontinent of bowel or bladder in front of their peers (other staff). I also thought about practices that really annoyed me, such as an uncovered catheter bag with urine in it or residents "parked" around the nurses' station so the staff can "keep an eye on them."

As the administrator, I felt the staff needed to know what it was like to trade dignity and choice for convenience and time.

These were all challenges that were easy to simulate by putting the program participants in some of these exact situations.

## Your Diagnosis Is . . .

In setting up the contest, we came up with diagnoses for participants to draw randomly out of a basket, such as the following: *You have a right hip fracture and are confined to a wheelchair. You are nonweight bearing along your right-lower extremity. You have confusion and try to get up without assistance. You must be kept in a supervised area when in your wheelchair or not in bed. You are not to be left unattended in the bathroom or during bathing.*

To come up with the initial diagnoses, we thought about some of the issues we were struggling with as staff, as well as the indignities our residents were experiencing because of our lack of knowledge and education in putting the diagnosis before the person. One reason why we chose to include this particular diagnosis was because of our automatic response to a person standing up from a wheelchair who is at risk of falling. We would hurriedly say, "No, no, sit down. We don't want you to fall," get the person seated in the wheelchair again, and then continue on our way to the next task because we were so busy. We were not thinking about *why* the person was standing up. And what about *you are not to be left unattended in the bathroom or during bathing*? Why is that as soon as a person moves into long-term care, modesty is no longer an option? Why do we assume a person automatically feels comfortable being seen naked and being bathed versus bathing him- or herself? What were we doing to foster independence rather than promote dependence?

We were looking for the answers to all of these questions and were eager to get started.

## How Will We Ever Pay for This?

All of the participants and their families, if available, were required to go through the admission paperwork with our Social Services department. This process was a real eye-opener for our staff as to all of the expenses that are a part of long-term care. Learning the differences in the pay sources of Medicare, Medicaid, and private pay can be confusing, especially in high-stress situations of suddenly needing rehabilitation or long-term care. Rarely do people plan ahead of time for when they may need long-term care. Typically it is an acute situation, and finances often have not been discussed ahead of time. Amy, one of our 2011 contestants, and her husband thought that maybe they should look into long-term care insurance. It scared them to think that even though they were young, what if something happened to one of them, like a terrible car accident, and long-term care was needed?

## What about My Clothes?

Everyone had to mark their clothes with their names. I remember Leah, one of our first contestants, saying to me, "I brought the crappiest clothes out of my closet because I didn't care if they got ruined in our laundry." The unfortunate thing about institutional living is that everyone's clothes are washed together in large industrial washers and dryers and at times items get damaged or go missing. If a person is accustomed to wearing certain items, as a contestant in the program he or she would now need to figure out a way to continue to make that happen in his or her new home.

## Who Will Be My Roommate?

The participants were required to room with a resident currently living in the nursing home. Most of the residents were really supportive of this, with the exception of one, Alice. She had diabetes and often blamed the staff for her blood sugars being out of control. We all knew Alice was snacking in her room all the time, even though she denied it. When a program participant, who happened to be a nurse, was designated to room with Alice, she came into my office complaining. No way was she having this nurse live with her. Her snacking secret would be out. It was the only control Alice still had in her life and she was not about to sacrifice it. Food, the experience of choosing what and when we eat, is a really important part of our lives, and so it is for our residents. And when so many other things in their lives seem out of their control, food and the experiences around it can become even more important for them.

## Daily Challenges

For the first day, I let the participants get settled into their new role of living a dependent life. Soon thereafter, I began to give them daily challenges to contend with in addition to their initial diagnosis. Every day, several times a day, I approached each participant with a basket of challenges to draw from, such as: *You are incontinent of bowel and/or bladder; You have to be bathed by staff; You need to change rooms; You were evaluated by speech therapy and they recommend thickened liquids at meals.*

As with the initial diagnoses, in coming up with the daily challenges we put in the forefront what we thought needed to change for our residents. For example, when an elder's favorite pair of pants go missing and she is anxious she may never find them or someone took them, what do we do? We ask all the staff to be on the lookout for the pants. Then that request gets passed on to other shifts several times. What are the chances that those pants will be found? To be honest, looking for missing pants is low on the list of priorities for most staff, even though having those pants back would bring relief and joy to the resident.

When one participant, Leah, lost her phone charger, she said, "That's it! That's the straw that broke the camel's back!" Because she lost her phone charger? In the world of long-term care, we might start a Behavior Tracking Sheet with "irrational behavior regarding lost small item." I am exaggerating, of course, but only slightly. Most of the resident "behaviors" we track are situational—that is, caused by us, the people who think they know what is best for our residents. Staff might deem a pair of missing pants a low priority and not worth a resident being anxious about, but finding them would make a world of difference to the resident.

Think about what you could not live without in your daily life. Would it be your favorite pillow or caffeinated coffee or maybe your cell phone charger? You determine and prioritize what is important to you, no one else. Nor should staff decide how important something should be to a resident. Think of your daily pleasures. Is it having a morning cup of coffee in quiet before the rest of the world around you is awake? Is it playing with your dog when you come home from work? What if these simple pleasures were taken away when you moved into a nursing home? Now, think of what you take for granted, like taking a shower by yourself or using the brand of shampoo you like or putting your shoes on and going for a walk outside whenever you feel like? Many of these choices are taken away from you when you move into a traditional nursing home.

The first group of staff to participate in Through the Looking Glass were all about to experience these losses. I wanted the initial diagnoses and daily challenges to have a big impact.

The staff moved in excited and nervous all at the same time. They really wanted to do this to learn more about what the residents go through, but they had no idea what kinds of challenges were waiting for them.

# 2

---·◆·---

# Meaning and Purpose in Our Lives

## Darlene's Story

*"My parents were in a nursing home and
I wanted to see what it was like."*

On Monday, November 2, 2009, Darlene moved into the nursing home. Every one of the staff members had a reason or a story as to why he or she chose to participate in Through the Looking Glass. Darlene's was because her parents had lived in a nursing home and she wanted to see for herself what it must have been like for them. She was one of our housekeepers at the time, and shared an interesting observation with me as another reason why she wanted to move in: "As a woman and a housekeeper here, I have wondered what it was like for women to care for their homes all their lives and to suddenly have that taken away."

In our own busy lives, we often say it would be nice to have someone take care of cleaning our home and doing the laundry for us. However, we all need meaning and purpose in our lives, and for many women taking care of our home is just that. *Meaning and purpose.* It is what we do. It is part of our identity. It is something we take pride in. Some of us hire someone to clean our home or do our laundry. There is a difference, however, between hiring someone to do those tasks because we no longer want to or do not have the time and hiring someone because we no longer *can* do those tasks. As human beings, we need to feel some sense of control. Having someone clean our home because we no longer can is giving up control. As care partners, we need to find a way to put some of that sense of power and control back into the residents' hands.

Let me give you an example. Everyone has a particular way they like to make the bed. Close your eyes and picture your own bed. Is your pillow underneath the bedspread or on top? Is the sheet tucked under the mattress tight on all sides or is it haphazardly out? Do you have a quilt folded at the bottom? Think about how important that bed is to you and the way you like it made. Maybe your spouse makes it differently than you do and it drives you crazy. Well, it drives our elders crazy, too. They have had to give up so much to come live with us—beautiful homes that were all their own—to live in a small, shared space where someone else is going to determine where their things should go and how clean or messy their things will be kept. I will tell you this, the most important thing in residents' rooms is their bed, and they want it made the way they are used to. Involve them in that decision and in that process. No matter how trivial you think it is, it is one of the few choices they have left.

Darlene's initial diagnosis was that she had a recent stroke and had paralysis along her left side. Some of her daily challenges were being incontinent of urine and having MRSA and needing to be in isolation, to name just a few. As part of her diagnosis, Darlene had to eat puréed food and be moved from her bed to a wheelchair with a mechanical lift. We simulated the paralysis by placing 3-pound weights and a sling on her left arm and leg. She could not move anything on that side.

After she got to her room, she said she was really nervous about her decision to do the contest. Unfortunately, none of us get to decide whether or not to have a stroke and to move into long-term care as a result.

Darlene's stay drained her both physically and mentally. By day two, she was in tears because of the pain she felt from not being able to move her left side. She did not quit, though. "Our residents can't quit, so I won't either," she said.

When she drew the challenge, *You have been incontinent of urine and your call light is not within reach,* she shouted, "Why am I getting the worst ones?" The worst ones, I thought? Some of our elders are incontinent of urine every single day.

We simulated the incontinence by pouring water on her clothes. I made her lie there for 30 minutes. I told her it was shift change and the staff had to get report from the nurses first before checking on her. "I'm sure they'll come check on you when they're done. They'll notice you've been incontinent, and they'll get you changed then," I said. Going back a few minutes later, I reassured her, "It shouldn't be much longer. They're coming."

After just three days, Darlene stopped combing her hair and putting her makeup on, things that were a part of her daily routine before moving into the nursing home. They became less and less important as the days went on. Even though her initial diagnosis and the daily challenges did not prevent her from combing her own hair and putting on her makeup, it was remarkable to see how quickly she quit caring about how she looked. This was the case for many of the participants. The fact that they could not do some things for themselves took over their mental and emotional states, so much so they even stopped doing what they still could do. It was learned helplessness.

Do you see this happen with residents in your own community or with a friend or family member you are caring for? Think about how quickly helplessness sets in when you are dependent on someone else for some of your basic needs. We see residents quit caring about doing anything for themselves, even if it is taking a shower or running a comb through their hair.

I asked Darlene during her stay what she missed the most about her life outside of the nursing home. "I miss my home," she said. "I miss my bed, my freedom. I miss having the energy to do things."

On day two, Darlene wrote in her journal:

> I got up for breakfast already having a bad day. I don't know if I can make it. Now I'm on isolation and have to wear a mask all the time. I went out to the living room and listened to music. I had to eat dinner in my room. My son came to visit me, but there's not much else to do since I'm on isolation, so I just stayed in my bed the rest of the night.

Living in the nursing home was essentially draining the life right out of her. Darlene was feeling helpless and hopeless, feelings she had not expected to have with this experience. It was only supposed to be about sitting in wheelchairs and eating puréed food. When did emotion decide to come creeping in?

Darlene wanted to go home.

I am sure many of you working in long-term care have had an elder say to you, "I just want to go home." I often tell our staff and families that it is not just the physical place "home" that the person is longing for, but also the independence and personal space that came with it. How often have you replied, "This is your home now. You live with us." Is that really what the person wants to hear?

Think about what home means to you: freedom, privacy, friends, family, love, control. Are you creating an environment where your residents can enjoy these important aspects of home? Think about what Darlene said about missing having the energy to do things. Are you creating a home full of meaningful engagement, or are people merely sitting around sleeping the day away? This does not mean you have to offer an activity calendar full of things to do every hour. Entertainment and engagement are two very different things. I can sleep through a rock concert if I am not engaged in the moment.

By day five, Darlene was ready to move out. At noon that day, she wrote in her journal:

> I had a hard time sleeping last night. My roommate had a machine that kept me up, and she was up going to the bathroom a lot. I didn't get to sleep until 2:30 in the morning. I ate breakfast and then drew my next challenge. It was a room change. The only room change I want is my room (at home). I give up. I don't really feel like I've given up. I just feel like I've had enough. I'll never forget what I did, but I never want to do it again.

After Darlene moved back into her independent life, she said it took almost a week to feel like herself again. In fact, she had felt depressed when she first moved out. There were so many factors that had played a key role in Darlene's mental state when she was living as a resident: depression, loneliness, and physical pain. Many of the participants said they had felt the same way. Their emotions went in many different directions, from feeling empty because their physical independence was taken from them to enormous feelings of guilt for having the privilege to just get up and walk away.

Darlene went from leading an independent and active life to having a life-altering event like a stroke that limited her physical mobility.

Even though she had some expectation of what was going to happen to her by participating in Through the Looking Glass, she was not mentally prepared for what it was going to do to her emotionally and physically. The constant focus on Darlene's negative outcomes made her feel that life in the nursing home was not worth living. She had to leave just to feel like herself again. In developing Through the Looking Glass, I was not prepared for just how difficult it was going to be on the staff and how quickly their positive attitudes would be extinguished.

# 3

· ◆ ·

# Maintaining Safety
# as well as Dignity

## Leah's Story

*"I hate my body alarm."*

WHEN WE BEGAN Through the Looking Glass in the fall of 2009, we were using personal body alarms on our residents to prevent falls. At one time, over half of our residents were wearing some kind of alarm. Think about that. About 40 people were attached to a box that monitored their movements. Some had multiple alarms, one for the bed and one for the chair. Imagine how much noise all of those alarms created.

One day, I was walking past a woman in her wheelchair, and she stopped me and said, "I can't move in my chair because this thing will go off." She had her hand on the string that ran between the clip attached to her sweater and the alarm box. We did that to her. It broke my heart. We made her anxious and afraid to move even the slightest inch because we were too afraid she would fall. We did not involve her in the decision to add the alarm to her wheelchair. Her safety was most important to us. Her dignity took a back seat. She was not a person. She was a fall risk who we needed to keep off the floor.

The concept of eliminating the use of the alarms was alarming itself. Many staff members believed that if we stopped using alarms, our residents would be constantly falling. One certified nursing assistant (CNA) went so far as to say that I must not care about our residents, that I must want them to fall. When I shared the story of the woman in the hallway who told me she could not move for fear of setting off her chair alarm, the staff sympathized with her but still felt strongly that her safety was more important. There was no way for them to know how she felt.

We slowly began to decrease the use of the alarms by first examining the amount of falls a person had had within a 3- to 6-month period. We were more willing to risk removing the alarm if a person had not fallen in several months.

Eliminating alarm use is a process. I would never suggest to any community that they eliminate them all together without putting another process in its place. For us, that other process was not a less-restrictive restraint, but rather our team digging deeper into what was actually causing the falls in the first place. We had to put the person before the task and stop using the alarms as a babysitter.

By the time the first two Through the Looking Glass participants had moved in, we had managed to decrease our alarm use to eight residents from about 40. While this was a huge accomplishment, we still had not eliminated their use entirely. We were still compromising the dignity of eight residents with this fall prevention practice. These last eight alarms became the focus of our first group of participants, each of whom had to live in the same room with a resident who wore a body alarm as well as wear a body alarm at times during their stay.

———◆———

Leah was working as a CNA at the nursing home and wanted to move in because, "It's a chance to realize what the residents experience on a day-to-day basis, and at the end I hope to become more empathetic."

She drew the following diagnosis: *You have congestive heart failure. You have a personal body alarm in bed and in your chair because you are weak and at risk for falling. You must be assisted to and from the bathroom and use a wheelchair for long distances.*

Leah moved in with an air of cockiness about what she was embarking on. She would zoom around the facility in her wheelchair with a this-is-easy sort of attitude.

Leah was the first participant who had to wear a body alarm. By the end of her first day, she learned that being that active in a wheelchair would not be quite as easy as she thought. Her alarm was constantly standing guard, monitoring her every movement and reminding her when she was moving in a direction she was not supposed to.

This restriction was reflected in Leah's first journal entry:

Day 1: The excitement of moving in and having all the employees come in to meet me made the day seem to fly by. After supper, however, the newness of the situation had worn off, and the reality of it all has begun to set in. I'm normally very independent and constantly occupying my time. Now, I barely move, and my alarm starts dinging. It's quite frustrating. I'm also having a hard time falling asleep. I'm accustomed to silence and pitch-black dark conditions.

After Leah's first night, she drew the challenge "Room Change." At first she was excited about this because her first roommate needed a lot of assistance at nighttime, which was interrupting Leah's sleep. But with her room change, she still had to deal with the sound of alarms:

> At first I was getting more sleep, but then my new roommate had bed pad alarms, and from 3:00 a.m. to 6:30 a.m. she was up in 20-minute intervals.

It did not take long for Leah to say that she hated her body alarm as well as her roommate's. Quite the change for someone who before participating in the program had thought it was a great idea to use alarms on the residents to keep them safe.

That morning, after a night with very little sleep, Leah said, "I can't imagine what it must be like to be wearing this thing if you have dementia. It must scare the crap out of them."

Of course it does! It also inhibits the residents from getting a good night's sleep, which puts them at an even greater risk of falls.

Could that be right? Using body alarms can actually cause falls? Yes, they can. Eventually, the staff became immune to all of the alarms going off. They could not possibly keep track of 40 alarms going off, and after so long we did not even hear them anymore. The amount of extra noise body alarms cause in your community wears on everyone who lives and works there.

Leah's roommate would often walk to the bathroom before a staff member could even get to her. Thankfully the roommate never fell during Leah's stay, but she did give Leah a colorful narration about how often the alarm sounded.

Leah was beyond exhausted and irritable by her third day living in the nursing home. She was not buzzing about in her wheelchair anymore. She would not even visit with her peers anymore.

That same day, she drew the following challenge: *I tried to get up on my own and fell. I hit my head and need to have neurological checks every 2 hours for 24 hours.*

Think about how little sleep she was getting. Our bodies do not function well on just a few hours of sleep at a time. Leah also was not eating much, which was putting her at an even greater risk for falls. Her mood was also diminishing.

I continued to push Leah with challenges, and the next afternoon she drew, *We lost your cigarettes.*

I heard Leah yelling in the dining room. She could not take it anymore! She had reached her maximum stress threshold. I took her back to her room so she could calm down. She did yoga stretches to relax, and, much to her relief, her grandmother brought her another pack of cigarettes.

At lunchtime on day five, she drew the following challenge: *Your clothes have been mixed up in the laundry and you are wearing someone else's outfit.*

That was Leah's breaking point.

"You really want me to wear someone else's clothes?" she asked with pleading eyes.

Leah packed her things and moved out that day. I could not believe that out of all the challenges she had been put through—body alarms, a room change, very little sleep, lost cigarettes—that this was her breaking point. She later explained to me, "I take care of that person and I know how incontinent she can be sometimes. Even though I knew the clothes were clean, I just couldn't make myself put them on."

With the practice of consistent caregiver assignments and specific interventions for the residents, we were able to eliminate personal body alarm use. At the time, we were the first community in our area to do so. It became such a big deal that I had to inform our hospital discharge planners that it was a practice we felt we could no longer justify. Some families chose our home for their loved one in part because we no longer used alarms, while other families were afraid to choose us because we were not using them. Eliminating their use became one of our first "nonnegotiable" practices. We felt so strongly about not using personal body alarms that we were willing to risk a family choosing not to have their loved one live with us. We also provided a lot of education to our residents, their families, our staff, and even the Illinois Department of Public Health surveyors.

If you are still using personal body alarms for fall prevention, ask yourself, "Are we doing this for staff convenience or to protect the resident?" This is a really tough question to face. It was a tough dose of reality for us as well.

Leah's roommate did not need an alarm for fall prevention. We only thought we were protecting her. Or maybe we were more worried about protecting ourselves. Sometimes you just have to live it to figure it out, which is exactly what Leah had done.

Fall reduction (notice I did not say fall *prevention*, because we will never prevent all falls) has to be a proactive approach. To be proactive, you have to treat the problem, not the symptom. Anticipating the needs of those we are caring for is really hard to do if you have not developed a close care partner relationship with them. This was a great lesson in transforming our culture away from being reactive to situations and adopting more proactive approaches. We no longer used the alarms to tell us when a person was about to fall or had already fallen. Eliminating the alarms forced us to communicate with each other as well as with our residents to get at the heart of what was causing the falls.

# 4

◆◇◆

# Being a Care Partner
# Instead of a Caregiver
## Chris's Story

*"I want to learn from the residents."*

CHRIS WAS THE THIRD participant to take part in Through the Looking Glass. When he moved in, he drew the diagnosis of having had a recent stroke. His speech was garbled, and he was restricted to a wheelchair. The stroke affected his left side, and he could not move his arm or leg. To make sure he would not move them, we strapped down his left arm and leg and put weights on them to feel like the weighted limbs of paralysis (as we had done with Darlene).

This was actually the diagnosis Chris was hoping to draw, and he immersed himself in this new role the entire time he lived in the nursing home. Why would he want to put himself through this? He was a young college student working as a CNA, and he was curious. He told me that when I proposed the idea of staff moving into the nursing home, his first thought was, "What could be so hard about wheeling around in a wheelchair all day and getting paid for it?"

As was Leah's experience, he soon learned it was harder than he thought it would be. After day one, Chris wrote in his journal:

> My leg is very sore from wheeling around yesterday. I thought it would be easy, but after a while, you start to lose energy fast.

It had only been 24 hours.

By his third day, he wrote:

> Being an active and energetic person, the toughest part of my day was just sitting around. I was either in bed or confined to my wheelchair. It hurts my bottom, my legs are very antsy, and not being able to move my left side most definitely takes a toll on the body. I just wanted to get up and move around.

Chris was bored. And he was sick of sitting in that wheelchair, but the staff thought it was the safest place for him. He just wanted to get up and move around and do the things he was used to doing. We are supposed to be able to use a wheelchair to take us places when we cannot walk. They are not meant to imitate a comfy lounge chair to watch TV in or become our chair at the kitchen table where we visit with friends and family. Take a look around your long-term care community. Notice how many elders are sitting around in wheelchairs. If where they are living is supposed to be home, then have them sit on a recliner, sofa, or big comfy chair. Who sits in a wheelchair at home to watch TV?

## "I'm not wiping your ass."

When I present Through the Looking Glass at conferences and workshops, a frequently asked question is how staff feel about having to take care of their co-workers who have volunteered to be a resident for an unknown number of days. I will let Chris tell you, because he revealed the honest and harsh truth in his journal:

> As a staff member, sometimes we complain about certain residents or things we have to do but don't want to. I never really had the chance to realize how it makes the residents feel. During the entire evening shift, none of the staff did anything for me other than get me out of bed and put my shoes on and tie them. Every time I spoke as a stroke patient, asked to go anywhere, or asked them to take me to the bathroom, they refused and just said, "Take yourself. You can do everything by yourself. All we have to do is Hoyer lift you out of bed only this one time, and then we don't have to mess with you."
>
> One time a staff member just pushed me into the bathroom from the outside, shut the door, and didn't even help me stand up. When I hit the bathroom light, for 2 minutes all I heard was staff arguing about how they're not going to go in there and get me.

In another entry, Chris wrote:

> I decided to go to bed a little earlier because my legs were very sore. I asked evening shift to help me transfer. She stood at the edge of the bed and said, "Ok, go to bed." I asked her to help me stand up since I can only use one side. She said, "No, go to bed." I got up slightly and lowered myself to the floor as if I fell, and she said, "I'm leaving in 2 seconds. Pick yourself up." Then she left.

What? I did not see this coming. It was so hard to read about how some staff had reacted to Chris. I was heartbroken and embarrassed that this was happening in *my* facility. I was so angry that some of the staff were working as hard against what we were trying to accomplish as others who were working for it. I mean, this empathy program was a great idea, was it not? How was it that not every single person who worked here felt the exact same way as I did?

Reality check. I realized this was my fault. I had been so focused on the outcomes of the participating staff and had spent very little time discussing the expectations of the staff who had to care for them. The staff who had agreed to participate in the program had volunteered to do so. They were making a choice to do so. The staff who had to take care of them? They had not volunteered. They were not given a choice. It just became a part of their job.

This setback did not become a reason to stop doing the program. Instead it opened up an opportunity for more communication about staff expectations and what everyone can learn from the program. I began to involve more staff in choosing challenges for the participants and asked more questions, such as, "I would like the participant to experience what it's like to have to be bathed in a common shower room. When is a good time for that to happen? Are you comfortable with that? How should we simulate this challenge?"

When I started to write this book, I pulled out Chris's journal and reread it. It was tough to relive who we were at the time. "Past tense, right?" I thought to myself. "We weren't those people anymore, were we?"

As Through the Looking Glass has evolved, I have seen with my own eyes our staff take care of their co-workers with the same love and compassion they show in caring for our residents. But I have also sensed the stress and frustration when it is a busy day and they have to take time to give their co-worker a shower. There have been growing pains, for sure, but they are a part of the journey of change.

Sometime during the first year of writing this book, Jessica, a CNA in our community since 1999, and I had talked about the growth of the program and how staff were reacting to taking care of their co-workers who were participating. I hoped, prayed, and kept my fingers crossed that she was going to tell me all of what Chris had shared in his journal was behind us. She said,

> It is, mostly. I think that our staff's outlook on it has really changed. We realize it's a learning experience for all of us, especially those participating, and we don't want to take that away from them. It's hard, though, when you have two call lights going off and one of them is a real resident and the other is not. Of course, we are always going to choose the real resident. We can see, though, how this might make the participants feel like they are a bother.

We talked about how we could make the program less intense for the nonparticipants. Jessica suggested not having everyone move in at the same time. "It just seems more hectic when they are all living here at the same time," she said.

Collaboration. I like that.

## "I don't want to be a bother."

Worrying about being a nuisance seemed to be a common thread of each participant's experience of Through the Looking Glass. Working in the community, the staff who became residents hated asking for help because they knew how busy everyone often was. I hear all the time from our elders, "I don't want to be a bother." If someone has fallen on the way to the bathroom and we ask, "What happened?" and an elder says, "Well, I didn't push my call light because I didn't want to bother anyone." Why are they so worried about bothering someone when they are paying thousands of dollars for us to take care of them? Is it because they hear the staff talking in the hallways about how busy they are? Are we discouraging them from asking for help when they see us zipping up and down the hallways like there is not a minute to spare?

How do we encourage our residents to ask for help when they need it while fostering independence at the same time? I think that can be achieved when you become a care partner instead of a caregiver. The term *caregiver* suggests dependency, and dependency can make a resident feel hopeless. Also, a dependent person can feel subordinate to a caregiver. The dependent person can feel as though he or she has no power and that the caregiver has all the power.

Think about the term *care partner*. It says, "We are in this together." We are connected. We trust each other to be there for one another when we are needed. We make decisions based on what is best for both of us. We are a team focused on the same goal. That goal may be as small as eating a hamburger from a favorite fast food restaurant or as big as wanting to dance at a granddaughter's wedding. Care partners work as a team to make goals, big or small, happen. Care partnering is a relationship.

## "I miss my family."

Chris wrote in his journal about a visit from his grandparents and how other residents shared with him how much they miss seeing their own family:

> My grandma and grandpa came to visit today and brought ice cream and crosswords to do. It was very nice talking to them. I noticed that some residents aren't as lucky. Some don't get any visitors at all. Jean and Mona would just love to be at home with their family for Christmas. Bill, another resident, said that just hearing from his family once a day is all he really wants.

During the time he did the program, Chris was also a part-time student. He had moved in over the Thanksgiving break to avoid missing classes. I can remember him asking me if he could go home to his family for Thanksgiving dinner. I reminded him of the rules of the program; his time away would be deducted from the total time he stayed. Chris went home for Thanksgiving, and later that evening wrote in his journal about how that made him feel:

> I was allowed to leave for Thanksgiving to eat with my family and relatives from out of town. Even though I was able to go, I felt very sad for the residents who had to stay or didn't have family to come visit them. Family and friends really make a huge difference and just make the residents happy. When you just watch TV or play a game, it has to be very depressing for them.
>
> There was a large group of people in the living room earlier in the day watching the Thanksgiving Day parade when I was talking to a resident. She said she was nervous because there was a lot of activity going on. When I asked her if she liked being with other people, she said yes, but a lot of the time she just gets really tired. She thanked me and squeezed my hand about 10 times just for taking the time to talk to her for 20 minutes.
>
> I already miss the good company of my family, and I've only been back at the nursing home for 2 hours.

One of Chris's goals for moving in was to have a conversation with every single resident. He wanted to feel connected to the elders as a friend and as someone with some commonalities. He wanted to build relationships with them, something he had not been able to do as their caregiver. As a CNA, always busy working, he felt like he never really had time to do this. He built a relationship with the woman he spoke with in the living room. He cared about what she thought about Thanksgiving. He wanted to hear about her favorite memories. He took the time to listen to her, and she listened to him. They connected and she thanked him by holding his hand for what seemed like a long time in Chris's mind—not because he minded, but because he felt like his time with her was so short and he was not deserving of so much love in return. Chris was building relationships, and relationships build community. And community is the antidote to loneliness. In that moment, Chris and the resident felt less lonely.

Chris decided to end his time as a resident after going home for Thanksgiving. The home-cooked meal, time with his family, and the taste of independence he had not had for the past week were the gravitational pull to say good-bye to dependent life.

His last journal entry before moving out sums up well his experience of Through the Looking Glass:

> Spending a week as a resident really opened my eyes. I didn't know what to expect. This competition was very hard physically, emotionally, and mentally. I think it would be very beneficial to others who are considering work in this kind of atmosphere. I feel that talking to residents and experiencing, firsthand, how the staff really treats residents at times will really help make people understand and be more compassionate. Being in a wheelchair, drinking thickened liquids, and every day challenges were hard, but I had no problem dealing with those things and feel like I could go a full 2 weeks as a resident because of my positive attitude and mind-set.
>
> I didn't decide to quit because I couldn't do it anymore, it was too hard, I was sick and tired, etc. I wanted to really experience life as a resident, and I've done that. I also talked to as many residents as I could for at least 30 minutes each, some even for over 2 hours. I felt like I really got to know them. They all talked to me about life in the nursing home and before they came here. They told me what they liked and didn't like to do. They gave me complaints about staff, the food, and their rooms. They told me about what they loved about holidays and different seasons. I've done my very best at writing it all down, as well as informing the CNAs and nurses to help the residents out.
>
> Even though I could continue to stay and just sit around and do nothing just to win, that's not what I came

to do. I want to learn from residents, and if I'm not doing that, then there's no point to just sit and be a vegetable for another week.

I've had a really great experience, and it definitely will help me to be a better CNA and nurse. I think it would be vey beneficial to other people thinking about coming into the field, and I would definitely do it again.

———•◆•———

Chris decided not to continue nursing school and instead became a certified occupational therapy assistant in long-term care. A few months after graduating, he said farewell to Aviston Countryside Manor and moved to Chicago, taking his experiences to the community where he now works.

I had the chance to check in with Chris and ask if participating in Through the Looking Glass still affects how he approaches his work. He said,

I feel the program has truly changed the way that I even look and speak with the elderly population. Before the program, even while I was a CNA, the residents at the nursing home were just residents. They were people that I worked with and took care of. In my line of work as a certified occupational therapy assistant, in order to perform my job, I need to get to know the people that I work with. I have to learn about their life, what they love, what they want to get back to doing, and what is stopping them from doing it. By going through the program, I feel like I am more able to truly get to know them and build a more-personalized treatment approach.

Chris took the time to see the person in each one of the residents he lived with. He valued what each one of them had to offer and learned life lessons that he will carry with him always. Through his experience, Chris became a care partner.

# 5

⸺ ·◆· ⸺

# Loneliness in
# Long-Term Care
## Katherine's Story

*"Loneliness does not come from having no people around you,
but from being unable to communicate the things
that seem important to you."*

—Carl Gustav Jung, Swiss psychiatrist and psychoanalyst

KATHERINE, OR "KAT," was the last of the first group in 2009 to move into the nursing home. Like Leah, Kat worked as a CNA at Aviston. She drew a diagnosis of congestive heart failure and was required to wear oxygen at all times. She also had to wear a personal body alarm and move from place to place in a wheelchair because she was too weak to walk.

Kat shared with me that during her stay she was overcome by a sense of loneliness. Her freedom of being able to go and do things whenever she wanted had been taken away. When Kat moved in, she had to leave behind her pets, who brought her much comfort. Without them with her, she lost the responsibility of caring for them and being loved by them in return, and she also lost a very deep purpose in her life.

What is loneliness? *Webster's* defines *loneliness* as feeling alone or isolated or being without companionship and support, all of which Kat had experienced when she participated in Through the Looking Glass. Similar to Chris, Kat immediately felt alone after moving in. She did not share anything in common with the people she was living with and was the only one in her situation, which made her feel isolated. And she did not have the support of her fellow co-workers or contest participants or the companionship of family and friends.

How do we combat loneliness in long-term care? Close your eyes and picture the community where you work. What do you see?

During one of my presentations about Through the Looking Glass to a group of long-term care professionals, including administrators, social workers, surveyors, and ombudsmen, I asked, "What makes living in long-term care lonely?" Some of the responses included less community interaction, drastic life changes, fewer family visits, and self-isolation due to hearing loss and decreased vision. Another person said, "Long-term care isn't lonely because the staff keep it lively." I wondered if that person had ever actually experienced living in the community she was referring to.

I then asked how residents combat loneliness in their communities, and received answers such as watching TV, doing crafts, listening to music, engaging in a pet therapy visit, going on outings, and participating in activities that engage the senses.

Answering the question, "What makes living in long-term care lonely?" is easy to answer. We all respond with solemn faces:

*Families don't visit.*

*People see nursing homes as depressing places, so friends stop coming.*

*Residents can't just leave and go shopping when they want.*

One day I asked Steve, a 56-year-old resident in our community, "Do you think it's lonely here?" He said,

> The nurses and CNAs have all the power, and that makes it lonely.

I was surprised by his response, and so I asked him why he felt he did not have control over his life. He said,

> When I have to ask them if they will take me to the bathroom, I no longer have control. They do. That makes it lonely.

There is much we as care professionals can do to address loneliness among residents, including the following:

*Schedule activities:* We all like to have things to do. We want to know what is going on, what our options are for the day. In long-term care, we (the staff) worry about people spending too much time in their rooms, right? Scheduled activities provide a means of socialization and connecting with peers. They also get residents out of their rooms.

*Create an environment of community support:* It is never too late to make new friends. Are we creating an environment where residents have opportunities to make connections?

*Support autonomy:* Encourage each resident's ability to exist without being dependent on others for everything. We take autonomy in our daily lives for granted. This is the one thing that would cause the most panic in me about moving into long-term care. I want to be able to make my own decisions and determine when I want privacy and when I want to be around people. I want to be in control of my own life and not put control in the hands of those, including family, caregivers, and professionals, who think they know what is best for me.

When family, friends, and care partners think they know what is best for a person and begin making decisions *for* the person, rather than *with* the person, the person can feel isolated and alone. Imagine what it must be like to feel that everyone is against you and no one is on your side. You would feel defeated, depressed, and left without meaning and purpose in this world. Autonomy is what we, as long-term care professionals, need to give back to the people living in our communities who, like Steve, think they do not have control over their lives and feel loneliness as a result. Let your residents have control of their day-to-day with the support of family, friends, and care partners.

# 6

❖ ◆ ❖

# Honoring Choices

*"[W]hen we are here, we need to make the time
all about them."*

It was February 2011 when our next group moved in. By this time, Through the Looking Glass had really gotten the attention of not only people in the community, but also within the greater long-term care community through presentations I had given at several conferences. Our crash course in empathy had also been featured in an article in *McKnight's Long-Term Care News*. This was all very exciting for us, and I wanted to spread the word even more.

The next group was made up of nursing staff with a combined total of more than 30 years of experience in long-term care and included Aviston's Assistant Director of Nursing (Amy), the Director of Nursing (Tara), and two CNAs (Nikki and Victoria). Amy and Tara, of course, had the most experience. What else did they need to learn? As with their co-participants and those who had participated in 2009, they did not know what it felt like to be on the other side—to be the one being cared for.

### "I want to remember why I came to work here."

Nikki's experience of Through the Looking Glass has always stood out for me as one of the most meaningful. She had been working at Aviston since 2001. At the time Nikki participated in the program, she was in her mid-20s and at a crossroads in her life. Our community had been the only place where she had ever worked.

The morning she moved in, I asked Nikki why she chose to participate. Her answer was remarkable: "I want to remember why I came to work here. I don't want to be here because it's just a job."

One of her journal entries during her stay explains what inspired her interest:

> About a year ago, I was talking with my director of nursing and she mentioned that I don't smile anymore when I come into work. She said that I used to smile all the time. It was just a short little comment, but one that stuck in my head and I continued to think about it. She was right. At some point, I lost my view on what I do and it just became a job. I did my 8 hours, did what I needed to get done, and went home. I started to realize that when I began working here 9 years ago, I knew more about my residents than I do now. I decided that Through the Looking Glass would be a good way to remember why and who we do this work for.

The program had been full of emotional moments for all of the participants. Some of them were "ah-ha" moments, and others exposed every fiber of emotion, leaving staff members crying and full of passion to do something about what they had learned.

Two of Nikki's more revealing moments bring us both to tears whenever we talk about them. Nikki had drawn the challenge that she had had a stroke during the night, this in addition to her original diagnosis of congestive heart failure. Her journal entry the next day recognizes the struggle for those residents who cannot move their own bodies and who, because they have no other choice but to rely on staff to move them, may be left to languish in their wheelchairs because staff are too busy to move them where they want to go and where they want to be:

> I'm very crabby today. It's just not a very good day. I did break down emotionally over lunch. I cried. It's very frustrating that I cannot move any part of my body besides my left arm, and I can only move my left leg a little bit. It's just a bad, bad day. I have a better understanding of those residents who cannot move themselves around and understand how important it is for us to take the time to help them propel their wheelchairs.
>
> Oh, and because of my stroke I'm on thickened liquids and a puréed diet! (Definitely not tasty.) Not looking forward to supper or any other meal, for that matter. Really hope my night and tomorrow get better.
>
> The upside? I got a visitor today, which was the highlight of my day.

Nikki's other powerful moment happened during lunch that day. She was sitting at a table with other residents, and I noticed tears streaming down her cheeks while she was eating her puréed food. I asked, "Nikki, what's wrong? Why are you crying?" She said, "This sucks. I had no idea it was going to be this hard."

What she said next, I will never forget:

> In a few days, I'm going to walk out of here because I will decide I'm done being a resident. I feel so guilty about that. Mimi, who really has had a stroke, doesn't get to do that.

Here, again, it is awful when you realize you *have* to depend on others to make choices for you, including not being able to eat whatever you want in whatever consistency you want it. There is no sugarcoating that. And it is okay to be angry. But as professionals, let us use that anger to fix what we can and give control back to those we are care partnering with.

Think outside the box. *Put yourself in their shoes.* Of course Mom does not want to eat the puréed food—would you? Let us work together to find a solution. But remember that working together means involving Mom in the discussion and honoring her choices. *Nothing about her without her.*

Nikki hated the puréed food. HATED IT. She could not wait to leave the nursing home and eat a Big Mac. She grew tired of feeling as though she was living on mashed potatoes and applesauce, and she had started to lose weight:

> For lunch, I once again enjoyed my mashed potatoes and pudding. I had the same for supper as well as applesauce. I was so excited to get that. I can't wait until I get to eat real food again! I've already lost 5 pounds, and I'm starving!

As an organization, we have talked a lot about puréed food and how we can improve the taste, texture, and appearance for our residents.

In the fall of 2014, Aviston began working with Carmen Bowman from Edu-Catering in conjunction with "The New Dining Practice Standards" report from the Pioneer Network. Our team has learned a lot about individualizing altered consistency diets. They do not have to be a standard, uniform diet. Each person's level of consistency is different. And a puréed diet does not have to mean all food is puréed. It can mean all food that you need or want to have puréed will be, but the food you do not want puréed or can handle in a different consistency will not.

For example, perhaps a resident could handle French toast cut up into very small pieces, but sausage has to be puréed. Every person is different, as well as everyone's level of progress. Just because a person is on a puréed diet does not mean he or she will always be on that diet. Maybe today a resident cannot handle French toast cut up into small pieces, and it has to be puréed. In a few weeks or months, however, that may change with close support from care partners.

If food has to be puréed, we need to make it look appealing to the senses. How many of us order something at a restaurant because we see it at another person's table ("Oh, that looks good. I think I'll order that."). Imagine if what you saw was puréed steak served in a bowl. It is still steak, right? You would never order it, though, because it does not look very appetizing or appealing.

We began experimenting at Aviston with food molds and made, for example, a puréed pork chop look like a pork chop. And for thickened liquids, we made smoothies and added natural thickeners, such as applesauce and yogurt, to enhance the flavoring and consistency.

The point is, food is so important in the lives of our residents. The entire experience of eating is more than just getting nutrition. Families and care partners should always strive to make the dining experience as individualized and fulfilling as possible. Our lives tend to revolve around where we eat, what we eat, and what time we eat. Let us always make dining an experience to look forward to.

On Nikki's fifth day living in the nursing home, I walked into her room with my video camera. She was in her bed with an oxygen mask to simulate congestive heart failure. The look on her face was one of dread because she suspected I was coming in to give her yet another challenge. What will it be this time? Incontinent of bowel? Room change? Or maybe she will have to have her co-workers, who are now her caregivers, bathe her?

Instead I asked her, "When you come back to work on Monday, assuming you'll no longer be living here as a resident, what do you think you're going to do differently?"

Nikki thought for a moment and then replied, with a sigh, "Slow down. Take more time with the residents."

That is why I started Through the Looking Glass.

Amen.

Best lesson EVER!

Nikki's last journal entry, after seven days living as a resident, summarizes her experience:

> This week has been very challenging, frustrating, emotional, and very, very eye-opening! I came into this not wanting to win, but to learn and remember. I definitely believe I have. I believe that this experience has changed me, and when I come back to work tomorrow, I will be making some changes in the way I go about my day. I'll take the time to sit and talk with my residents and build stronger, trusting relationships with them, something that will help me take better care of them. This was a very good experience. One I would strongly suggest others take part in as well.

By participating in the program, Nikki's passion was reignited. In fact, she continued to work at Aviston. How many people can say that they have made career choices based on how passionate they are about their job? How many are willing to make a change based on the inability to find that passion? I applaud Nikki for being willing to take that chance. And I was so humbled by her commitment.

## "It is very lonely in my room by myself."

Each first day of Through the Looking Glass starts out the same way—we meet in the conference room and talk about why everyone wants to participate, what their goals are, and what they hope to get out of the experience. Then, I pass around the basket and everyone pulls, at random, a diagnosis.

Amy's diagnosis was particularly challenging: *You have MRSA of the sputum. You become agitated easily and often pull off your mask, so you need to stay confined to your room. Visitors must wear a mask in the room. You are legally blind. You cannot see to read or watch TV, but can have the TV on so you can listen to it.* [To simulate the blindness, she had the TV covered at all times.]

The other participants giggled nervously. "Oh no!" they said through their laughter.

"I'm so glad that wasn't me," they whispered to themselves.

"That's gonna suck," Amy whispered.

"I'll trade you," another participant offered.

"No. You can't trade diagnoses," I told them. "Imagine how many people who live here who would love to trade, even for a day, what they have to live with all the time."

In their first 5 minutes of day one, the group already had a lesson in empathy.

In her first journal entry, Amy tries to put her diagnosis into perspective:

> Well, my day didn't start out too good, beginning with the diagnosis I pulled. I am blind and positive for MRSA of my sputum. This places me on respiratory isolation and I am confined to my room, which is hard for me, being an energetic person. It is very difficult being confined to such a small space to pace back and forth from my bed to the chair. It's almost exciting when I have to use the bathroom because I have somewhere to go.
>
> I am able to have visitors, but they are required to wear a mask when entering my room. Of course, being blind, it makes it difficult because I can't see a darn thing. It is very lonely in my room by myself. I am lucky to have friends that come visit me, but it makes me empathize

with those whose only visitors are the staff. The first day is always the longest, I am adhering to my surroundings and look forward to what tomorrow brings.

On Amy's second day, she felt the worry of not wanting to be a bother to staff, which so many residents themselves feel:

I made it through Day 2. I woke up bright-eyed and bushy-tailed, eagerly waiting for breakfast at 6:00 a.m. It's difficult knowing both sides of the spectrum. Since I didn't particularly enjoy supper, I was hungry first thing this morning. I knew that the staff was busy, so here comes the dilemma—do you ring your call light and ask for breakfast? Or do you wait until everyone else is up and it's not a pain in the butt for them to get your room tray?

The realities of the cost of long-term care also started to settle in for Amy:

Today, my husband came and filled out admitting paperwork for me. It's definitely an eye-opener realizing how much it costs to live here. You almost feel as if you could save your whole life and still never have enough.

According to LongTermCare.gov, the average cost to live in long-term care in 2012 was $62,050 per year. By 2037, it is projected to be $147,349 per year. This cost is based on a semi-private room in the state of Illinois. According to this same website, the average length of stay is one year. We probably all know of someone who has lived in long-term care for much longer than one year. With all of the money being spent on long-term care, you would expect to get good care. Each staff member who participated in Through the Looking Glass commented that he or she had no idea it was so expensive and felt the residents deserved the best care for their money.

After he completed the paperwork, Amy's husband said to her, "What if something like this really did happen to one of us? It makes me really think about how we would pay for it."

---

Two of the daily challenges I gave Amy taught her how difficult it can be for residents to deal with incontinence:

> My first challenge of the day: I was incontinent of urine in my bed, my call light was not within reach, and I had to wait until staff came by to check on me. At first it was warm, not bad considering in my mind it was still "just water." Then it got cold, almost sticky. My clothes stuck to my skin all the way from my mid-back to my knees. That's when it got uncomfortable. The realization hit me that some of our residents are like that often, whether they cannot make it to the restroom in time or they just cannot determine when they have to go. After I was cleaned up, I still ended up taking a towel to wipe all the way down my legs because I felt wet for quite a while after.
>
> Second challenge of the day: I am using a bedpan for urinating for the rest of the evening. I almost feel like I have to aim not to shoot it over the edge and wet my bed. I can definitely see how placement plays a major role.

I pushed the indignities with this group even more than I had with the first group. They had to use bedside commodes, be weighed in front of the other residents, and be bathed by staff—all things that we expect our residents to do without giving it a second thought. The truth is these can all be humiliating experiences for residents, which this group learned firsthand.

Think about how you would feel if you were asked to sit on a chair scale in a hallway in front of your neighbors and your weight was announced for all to hear? It is a very task-oriented practice that is done for staff convenience and without thinking at all about the residents. No matter where they were or what they were doing, they were weighed right then and there. No choice. No privacy. We eventually stopped bringing the weight chair around to everyone. It was an undignified practice.

## The Director of Nursing Moves In

Staff at every level were encouraged to participate in Through the Looking Glass. Having Tara, our Director of Nursing, move in was a particular source of pride for me. It showed everyone how committed our community was, including at the administrator level, to understanding our residents' experiences of living in long-term care.

Tara's journal entry from her fourth day is very telling:

> Day 4! It has been a very long 4 days for me. I have spent nearly half of the last 2 days in bed. It's been so boring. Yesterday afternoon I had an unresponsive spell and had to be put on bed rest until this morning around 9:30. I had to have supper last evening and breakfast this morning in bed. Some would think that's heaven, but I'm really not a fan.
>
> I also had to use the bedpan during that time, and I have one word to say about that—YUCK! I could not imagine losing the ability to toilet myself. First, I was afraid I was going to overshoot the bedpan because I waited until I really had to go. The other fear was overflowing or the urine spilling into the bed. Thank goodness my husband was here to help take the bedpan out from under me. Not at all a pleasant experience for him. He actually said, "to hell if someone else would help me do this." Unfortunately, our residents don't have that choice in most situations. They depend on us to provide for them.

> So, this morning's challenge placed me in a wheelchair
> with a catheter drain bag hanging from it for the world
> to see. How undignified! Then, lo and behold, right out
> in the living room was actually a resident whose drain
> bag was hanging under his wheelchair UNCOVERED.
> The worst part about it was that there was also a drain
> bag cover hanging under his wheelchair, but no one had
> taken the time to place the bag in the cover.

Tara's family visited so often that she felt like telling them to stop coming because it made it easier for her to stay and made her stay feel less lonely. Tara knew that the majority of our residents do not have family members who are able to visit daily.

Family visits made it easy, but losing control over taking care of her basic needs made Tara's stay very difficult. *"I cannot imagine losing the ability to toilet myself"*—this was a strong statement coming from a seasoned long-term care professional. Every day, Tara, along with all of us, see how dependent almost every resident is on staff to take them to the bathroom. It is one of the most common reasons a person makes the decision to move into long-term care.

Tara knew that. It was not a surprise to her. But being faced with that dependency herself struck her and changed how she viewed that dependency. It is not just a little thing that a person living in long-term care just has to accept and get used to. It is a big thing. It is like giving up that last piece in you that can say, "I am independent."

Here is a small exercise you can try in your own community to shed light on this challenge. Have the staff ask each other, "Can I go to the bathroom? Will you take me to the bathroom?" Then have staff members escort other staff to the bathroom. It sounds silly and feels silly, but it will put the challenge into perspective a little. It is not natural to have to ask to use the bathroom, and as care staff we should not downplay being dependent on others for what we view as a simple activity and one we take very much for granted.

Tara was also given the challenge to sleep for the night in a geriatric chair, or geri-chair, at the nurses' station. This had become a convenient practice for staff to keep an eye on residents who were restless and who staff were afraid would fall out of bed.

Tara wrote about her terrible night of sleep, but also reflected on how to change the practice:

> Well, the nurses' station setting is not conducive to getting any rest. Amy, Nikki, and Victoria kept me company until I decided to go to sleep at about midnight. With the fluorescent lights right above my head, I took the mask I was supposed to be wearing over my mouth (for MRSA of the sputum, yet another challenge) and put it over my eyes to try and eliminate some of the brightness. We sometimes place our elders, who may keep trying to get out of bed, at the nurses' station so that we can keep a closer eye on them. This is definitely not the place to try and get them to go back to sleep. A better idea might be to make sure all of their needs are met, such as hunger, thirst, and toileting. Then, try and sit with them until they go back to sleep. This may require more staff time, but I think in the end it would be a much more pleasurable experience and have better outcomes. Needless to say, I think I may have gotten about 2 hours of sleep all night.

Of note is that we do not even own geri-chairs anymore, and with ongoing education with new staff we have stopped the practice of "parking" residents at the nurses' station. We replaced the geri-chairs with real furniture, like recliners and comfortable chairs and ottomans. Real life. Real living.

# And Then There Was One

Of the group, Tara and Victoria were the last ones to end their time living as dependent residents of long-term care. On day 8, Tara decided to end her stay. "Victoria needs the money more than I do," she joked. "Besides, I already feel like a winner," she added.

Tara was ready to get back to work where she was needed, and it felt good and meaningful to her to be needed.

Victoria had won the challenge, and her final journal entry I think spoke for the entire group in expressing all that she had taken away from the experience:

> What a journey!
>
> Well, I am the last one standing. I have learned so much, but it's hard for me to put everything into words. I have learned that communication is very important. You may never hear a certain person talk unless you actually talk to him or her. When feeding the residents their meals, ask what they would like to drink, ask what they would like to eat, tell them what exactly they are eating, ask if it is too hot or too cold, and ask if they would like some more or something else. There is so much that could be asked, instead they just sit there and get what they get. That's just during meal times. Some residents don't get asked to go to activities, and they sit there bored, staring into space, waiting for the next meal to come around so they actually have something to do. It is such a simple task that just doesn't get done as often as it should. Talk to them. ASK them what they want.
>
> I hope to come back to work as a better CNA. I hope that I can encourage other CNAs to just take the time to give the residents what they really want. Too many people are focused on getting what they need done within a certain time limit or making sure they get to have their cigarette breaks and time to eat. I'm sorry, I don't even care if I get a 30-minute break. I don't even care if I get a 5-minute break. We are here for these

residents. We have all the time to ourselves when we leave this building, so when we are here, we need to make the time all about them.

Through the Looking Glass is about teaching staff empathy, and one overall lesson this group learned was the importance of honoring choices. Until you walk the walk, you truly have no idea what it is like to have staff decide when you will wake up, when you get your breakfast or dinner, or where you will sleep. Each of the challenges this group dealt with made them reflect on how they were doing their jobs and whether they were honoring resident choices.

For example, as I mentioned earlier, we talk a lot about mealtime in our community, because it often feels hectic, rushed, and very task-oriented. Get the meal out. Get everyone fed. Get everyone back to their rooms and toileted. That is the medical model of mealtime. Does this sound familiar? It is an example of a staff-centered practice (as with using chair scales and geri-chairs or having residents sleep near the nurses' station) that is difficult to move way from and instead create a more social and relaxed atmosphere driven by resident choices.

Our mealtime improvements started with breakfast. We committed early on in our culture change journey that we needed to stop waking people up if they were not ready to get up. This was a problem when breakfast was served at 7:00 a.m. only, but we expanded the breakfast hours to be from 6:30 a.m. to lunchtime. We also created choice in what a person would like to eat for breakfast by essentially becoming a short order kitchen in the mornings. For lunch and dinner we offer two different entrées, and everyone orders from a menu. And I do mean *everyone*, even those with cognitive impairments and those on modified diets. Everyone has a choice, which has created a lot more satisfaction among residents.

These changes have had a positive impact on multiple levels. What we call "behaviors" decreased. Our residents are getting more sleep, which generally makes them feel a lot better. If a resident with dementia is "combative with care" at 6:00 a.m., then we let the person sleep. There is no more "save her breakfast." Breakfast is still going on whenever the person is ready to wake up and eat. Life goes on as the person was used to at home. This approach has made so much more sense. A person's mind and body need sleep, which we had not been supporting by waking everyone up on our schedule. Think about it this way: each participant in Through the Looking Glass is exhausted by the end of his or her stay. This is also what we were doing to our residents.

This transition took some getting used to, and there has been an important key factor to our success in honoring residents' choices: every single team player—nurses, housekeepers, laundry staff, activities professionals, care partners—had to learn flexibility. They had to wear it like a badge of courage, because flexibility is not easy in long-term care. It takes bravery because we assume it is risky to veer off schedule and stop certain practices. Once you do it, however, it is like putting on your slippers the minute you get home from work— so much more comfortable.

Slow down. Take the time to listen to what your residents want. They make choices every day. We just have to be open to honoring them.

Slow down. When you begin honoring choices, like allowing natural waking times, the rhythm of your day, as well as theirs, will change. Trust the choices your residents make. It is their lives. Let them be the drivers.

# 7

⸻ ◆ ⸻

# What's Going to Happen to My Body Next?

*"I hope I can make their today and
their tomorrow a good one."*

BOBBIE, LORI, AND NATALIE together moved into Aviston in April 2012.
I decided to challenge this group a little differently. With the previous groups, the challenges that were randomly drawn (incontinence, being fed by staff, eating puréed food) did not necessarily follow along with the person's original diagnosis. With this group, each person's condition would decline as her stay continued, and the challenges she would draw would be based on her original diagnosis. I felt this approach would more realistically mimic our residents' experiences and that the participants would learn more from their stay as a result.

⸻ ◆ ⸻

Bobbie, Aviston's Life Enrichment Coordinator, drew the most difficult diagnosis. She had to live as though she had end-stage cardiac disease and was faced with the decision of whether to receive hospice care. She chose hospice and described in her journal the experience of her first two days after moving in:

(Day 1): I am so weak that I cannot get out of bed. I receive my meals in bed and have to use a bedpan.

I was admitted into hospice care today. The folks who have handled my admission have been very informative and have answered my questions.

I haven't enjoyed lying in bed all day. It has been exhausting. I have had visitors today, but nobody stayed very long. I am looking forward to my husband visiting this evening.

Using the bedpan has not been my favorite experience thus far; in fact, it has been a low point on my timeline. I hope it becomes, if not easier, neater. The oxygen cannula is making my nose itch and makes me want to sneeze. A lot.

I am amazed at how our elders get any rest here. Lying here I can hear a lot of life going on up and down the hall. Not that anyone is noisy; it's just an accumulation of sounds that makes it difficult to nap. I hope it will be quiet tonight so I can sleep some.

(Day 2): Last night and this morning I woke up, and woke up again, and woke up yet again to move and change position as my joints and muscles protested my inactivity of the day before.

I tried to use the bedpan again this morning, but my body was having none of it. Thank goodness I am having a good day and can get into a wheelchair to go use the toilet. I was able to spend some time out in the living room this morning. The residents and their families did double takes as they saw me in a wheelchair with oxygen, my PJs on, and my hair looking slept on. It is difficult to spend a lot of time in one place or another if you can't move on your own.

My body still protests my inactivity. I fear I am becoming constipated since I am normally very regular and have so far not been. I don't want to intervene, but nature so far has not taken its course.

My weakness grows and my diet has been downgraded to soft and easy-to-chew foods. Supper will be a new adventure. I will dare to shower tomorrow morning. I am treating today like a lazy Sunday and will stay in my PJs.

Bobbie did finally take a shower, but with the assistance of a CNA because of her weakness. The experience was awkward for her. As I mentioned earlier, it is not natural to give up control of doing something so personal, and we as long-term care staff cannot just assume that the people we are caring for are automatically okay with being naked in front of us. They are not. People do not box up their dignity and put it in storage when they move into long-term care. Honor their dignity. Respect it. Please.

Bobbie shared with me that being in hospice care did not have an emotional impact on her until she decided she wanted to end her three-day stay. Many of the people she had grown close to, who were in hospice, flashed through her mind. "The majority of the time, our residents on hospice don't have the opportunity to go home," she said. It felt eerie for her to decide to just leave, knowing that those in hospice are, sadly, nearing the end of life.

Lori was an occupational therapist contracted by Aviston Countryside Manor. She too wanted to experience what it is like to be dependent on others. As an OT, it can be easy to jump to conclusions or make assumptions about why a person may not be motivated in therapy. Surely they *want* to go home. We cannot know the emotions a person is going through until we experience them ourselves.

Lori's diagnosis was a right hip fracture. She was confined to a wheelchair and could not bear weight on her right lower extremity. Because of periods of confusion, she had to be supervised when she was in her wheelchair and could not be left unattended in the bathroom or during her showers. Much like the residents she worked with, Lori was afraid to use her voice, afraid to ask for help, afraid to speak her needs.

Last night wasn't quite as easy as I'd expected. I did not get to bed until around 11:00, which is when the CNAs came to get me for bed (I didn't get to choose my bedtime). I was so tired, but it took me a while to get to sleep (just not used to a twin bed with extra layers for my incontinence). The CNAs asked if I wanted my roomie's television turned down. I said no since it is her room and if she likes it that loud, I did not want to mess with her routine. But as 1:00 a.m. rolled around, and I had maybe slept for 20 minutes, I was regretting my decision to not turn it down. The TV continued to blare all night as I went in and out of sleep. I woke up at 5:30 a.m. to my roommate getting some meds from the nurse. Even though I was awake at 5:30, nobody got me up until my physical therapist came in at 7:15 a.m. (I am supposed to be confused and couldn't find my call light to tell them I needed to get up.) Thank goodness for the wonderful therapists, who got me up and ready for the day (with the help of my wonderful fiancé and some caregiver education).

I ate all of my breakfast and felt ready to tackle the day—until I drew my first challenge of the day. I became incontinent and had to sit with really cold water all over my pants at the nurses' station in my wheelchair. I kept trying to get up, but nobody ever asked me what I needed, so going to the bathroom right there was my only option. I definitely will ask residents more often now if they need to use the restroom. It was slightly embarrassing to sit there in wet pants. My wonderful CNA, Jennia, helped me change my pants.

My mom visited around lunchtime, and it was so good to see her and laugh with a familiar person who understood me. I was sad to see her go, but I looked forward to my fiancé and a co-worker visiting me this evening. I was given my second challenge of the day. My glasses became lost for several hours. I couldn't see clearly to read or look out in the hallway from my bed where I was resting. I got very dizzy, so I decided to take a nap. I don't usually take naps, so this tells you how bored and lonely and dizzy I felt without being able to see. BUT, I did take a shower without my glasses and with help from my occupational therapist. It was difficult to see what I was doing in the shower and getting out. I felt like a new person after the shower and realized how important it was for the residents to get showers more often. I will definitely try to incorporate working on the shower goals more often when I get back to work. This evening, I played bingo. It helped pass the time, but I had a lot to drink and need to use the bathroom—off to see if I can get my CNA to help me in the bathroom!

Feeling okay at the end of day two. I sure do miss my bed and family, but I feel like I definitely learned a lot today.

I remember the incontinence challenge that Lori wrote about. She was sitting at the nurses' station, and I poured water on her to simulate being wet with urine. Not even a minute had passed before Jennia, her care partner, asked me if she could take Lori to be changed. "No," I said. "I want her to be wet in front of others for a few more minutes." I could see the anxiety start to build up in Jennia. It had not dawned on me until that moment that this was no longer who we were. We were no longer a community that waited for a person to be incontinent, but instead a community that *promoted continence.* We had reached a level of empathy, compassion, and honoring a person's dignity that I prayed would happen as a result of Through the Looking Glass and all of our efforts to change our care practices. The incontinence challenges were for the staff, both the participants and nonparticipants in the program, to see how undignified it was to be soaked with urine and thereby understand the importance of checking in with residents more often to ask if they need to use the bathroom and recognize more quickly when someone needs to be changed. With this knowledge, we successfully decreased the level of incontinence among our residents over time.

⎯⎯•◆•⎯⎯

As with Lori, and before her Darlene (a member of Aviston's housekeeping team), participating in Through the Looking Glass has not just been for nursing staff. Natalie, Aviston's office manager, took on the challenge as well. She drew a diagnosis of congestive heart failure.

One evening during Natalie's stay, a resident asked her, "What's your diagnosis?" When she told him, he said, "That's what I have," and he began to tell her what to expect as her condition declined. Even though she knew her diagnosis was not real, she felt scared and worried. She later told me that when she saw me coming with the basket to draw a challenge, she became anxious and asked herself, "What's going to happen to my body next?"

At the end of her stay, when she recalled that moment, tears came flooding out of her eyes. It was significant to her to realize that our residents are real people dealing with real challenges every day.

Natalie, the winner for this group, had the shortest stay of all our winners (four days). But her short stay did not minimize the impact she felt. Reading her final blog post, I was so touched by how the experience took hold and made her stop and really think about our residents and what role she could play in their day to day:

> I was a little nervous when it was time for my interview after deciding to leave. Did I learn enough? It was barely four days. I have written about all the little things that seemed hard and complicated with the stay and my diagnosis. What was the one thing I was going to remember most? It hit me like a brick wall when Leslie asked me, What did you learn?
>
> One night, when I was sitting at the nurses' station, a resident with congestive heart failure came up and visited with me. He asked, "Have you had a water pill yet? Have your kidneys started to shut down? Are you on dialysis?"
>
> I did not think much of it at the time, but later started to worry about what was going to be my next challenge. That's when it hit me.
>
> We have residents who are at all stages of diseases. Every day, they see people who are at worse stages than they are with the same disease. Every day they are reminded of what is going to happen next.
>
> They cannot escape it.
>
> They go to bed every night wondering, "Am I going to be as bad as he is when I wake up? Am I going to wake up? My neighbor down the hall did not wake up yesterday."
>
> That has to be scary. Unfortunately, this is one thing I know I cannot change for our residents. But after this experience, I hope I can make their today and their tomorrow a good one.
>
> How am I going to do this?
>
> I honestly think it will be different for each person, but I am going to try.

Natalie, Bobbie, and Lori walked away with valuable lessons they were ready put into practice, which is a commitment I hope each participant feels inspired to take on. I encourage everyone not to let their experience be just their individual experience, but to teach and share with others what they learned.

Natalie does not have a direct caregiver role, so she does not always feel comfortable suggesting to a CNA of 15 years a better way to do something based on her experience of having lived as a resident. She does, however, have a unique role in being able to speak to brand new staff early on and ended her stay ready to share with them what she learned. It is at those moments engaging with new staff that she seizes the opportunity to share her experience of Through the Looking Glass and talk about the honor and respect that go along with not only working in long-term care, but also working in *our* long-term care community.

# 8

• ◆ •

# Every Resident Has a Voice

## All for One and One for All

CHELSEY, JENNY, AND BRIDGETTE lived in the nursing home for 10 days during the summer of 2013. Of all the groups to move in together, these three could not have been more different in where they were in their lives, and yet they also shared things in common. They had three very different personalities, but were very competitive. The challenges they were given created a lot of stress for them, but they were all stubborn. No one wanted to be the first to go. I put them through a lot, but nothing was enough to make them move out.

Bridgette and Chelsey were only 18 years old. They had graduated from high school just a few weeks prior to moving in. I cannot think of many recent high school grads who would want to spend part of their summer break, before starting college, living in a nursing home. Bridgette was working as a CNA, and Chelsey worked in the kitchen. Jenny was married and a very busy mom of three children. She worked at Aviston as a unit aide. I am in awe of these women when I think about the personal sacrifices they each were willing to make to participate in Through the Looking Glass.

I really pushed this group. They were bedridden for several days and had to use bedpans. I even asked their families to stop visiting for a few days. One of them was not allowed to use her voice to communicate. Another had to be blind, which she simulated by wearing goggles masked with tissue.

As with each time we invited people to participate in the program, we wanted to have a goal in mind of where we felt we needed to grow as a community in adopting a person-centered approach to care. The goal for this group was for them to recognize that every resident has a voice and can make choices in just about every situation, no matter his or her disability or health challenge.

## "The little things are the most appreciated."

Chelsey drew challenges for bed rest and of the three had to spend the most time in bed. She blogged about her experience, from how lonely she felt being confined to her bed to how the simple, everyday things in life are difficult for those whose mobility is restricted to how she would not have lasted as long as she did if not for visits from her family and friends.

### Chelsey (Day 1)

I arrived at 9:00 a.m. with my father and was admitted to the nursing home. My diagnosis: blind, C. difficile infection, and incontinent. I'm wearing goggles on my face and a diaper for my incontinence.

I came out and visited with other residents for a while. Then I played card flip. Deb, my care partner, assisted me back to my room. A friend came to visit me and we ate lunch together in the dining room. She brought me back to my room and we talked until I became sleepy, so I took a nap.

Leslie came to my room and woke me for my first interview on camera. I pulled a challenge that made me sit in pudding for 10 minutes to simulate the watery diarrhea from the C-diff. The CNAs had to change me and got me up out of bed. Afterwards, I watched a little TV, my father came for a short visit, and then it was time for supper.

Supper was a little slow tonight, but it tasted good. Emily visited me, and we played bingo. I won chocolate chip cookies. Then my mother came to visit for a while.

Overall the day was not too bad. I did not enjoy the pudding or the cleanup. Walking around with the goggles is a challenge.

### Chelsey (Day 5)

I woke up and began my day with breakfast in bed. Breakfast in my room was a quiet and lonely experience. With the assistance of an aide, I took a shower. It is amazing how these simple things we do every day are so difficult when you have a disability. I was able to sit in a wheelchair but needed the assistance of someone else to maneuver me around the halls and my room. The nurse helped me with exercising my muscles to keep them strengthened.

I was able to play cards with a resident. Interacting with everyone that lives here is a wonderful experience. It was great to be able to eat lunch with everyone in the dining room. Afterwards, I was asked to label my clothes so they could be laundered. My friends visited, and they strolled me around the building in a wheelchair. When I returned to my room, it was time for another challenge.

The new challenge was that I reinjured my left hip, which meant wearing 20 lbs. of weights on my left leg.

I also fractured my right arm and now must wear a sling at all times. Due to these injuries, I am on strict bed rest with an abductor wedge in between my legs. I must also rely on staff for all toileting needs and use a bedpan if necessary. Due to my bed rest, I was forced to have dinner in my room.

That is so lonely. I remained in my room, with an unpleasant roommate, the rest of the night. My roommate was tired and informed my visitors that they had to leave immediately because she was going to bed at 7:00 p.m. One of my co-workers also tried to visit after her work hours (8:00 p.m.) and was forced out. I feel that my quality of life is slowly fading away.

## Chelsey (Day 10)

Today is day 10! Staff woke me up and I could not go back to sleep. I began my day with breakfast in the dining room. I was bored and asked the housekeeper if she needed something to be done. So I helped wipe down all the side rails. I didn't feel helpless anymore. I felt helpful and important. Afterwards, I was given the challenge of eating puréed food for the rest of the time that I was planning on staying here. I didn't like this challenge because I serve this food to the residents, and it does not ever look appetizing. I took my first bite of the puréed pork chop, and it was so gross, so all I had for lunch was a bowl of pudding. I then got emotional and began to cry because some of the residents only get to eat puréed food every day, and I felt bad for them. I am also really missing my parents and my house. I am tired of being treated like a resident and want to go home. My father came to visit, so we sat outside. I've realized that most of the residents don't get visitors every day. I would hate that. Without my visitors, I would not have lasted as long as I did.

I got to play bingo that night and won a quarter. Everyone gets so excited when they win. It's a reminder that the little things in life, like winning a quarter, are just as important.

I would have never thought this would be my last day of living in the nursing home! I enjoyed living here and enjoyed getting to know what the residents actually have to deal with every day. I've learned that being a resident is not easy. I've learned that all the little things are the most appreciated. I've also learned that we need to be patient with the residents and not just do the job just to get it done. We should be more caring and understanding to the residents because they have problems too, and we should listen to them.

## "Does anyone care I'm in here?"

Jenny's diagnosis was congestive heart failure. She had to use a wheelchair to move around. Throughout her stay, we placed weights on her legs and chest to simulate the heaviness of the fluid building up in her lungs.

### Jenny (Day 3)

Today brought about many emotions. I did not have much sleep last night. It felt as though my legs had been tied to the bed, and I was unable to move. There was no way to get comfortable. Trying to move while asleep just woke me up. At some points, it almost brought me to tears, even though I have a high tolerance for pain. Is this how a lot of the residents feel every day? Sometimes, we wonder why a resident is in a bad mood or crabby. Walk towards those people who are crabby. If they are hurting, like I have been, it's understandable. My advice is give an extra pillow for their legs and back or adjust the bed in a better position to try to help relieve some of their discomfort.

My first challenge was to be showered and have my teeth brushed by an employee. I see and work with these people all the time, yet I was very self-conscious about it.

I also felt worthless. It was a moment when I realized, again, just how much we take little things for granted and they mean so much.

My next challenge was to stay in bed and have lunch in my room. What a lonely place. You can see the sun, but you can't go outside. There are activities where you'd see people you know, but you're not able to go. There's no TV to watch and no one to talk to. It's depressing. You wait and hope someone will come in to see you. When no one does, your mind wanders to thinking "Does anyone care I'm in here?"

My night challenge is to sit up in bed and sleep. I watched my dad do this for years. I know his back hurt from it and I'm prepared for it, too.

The highlight was seeing my family. Knowing they were coming lifted my spirits.

Tomorrow's a new day and I look forward to whatever comes my way.

### Jenny (Day 4)

To my surprise I did not wake up in the pain I thought I would have from sleeping sitting up. It was a matter of finding the right position, and it was a better night of sleep. After breakfast, I went and sat under the overhang near the front door to the "house." There was a storm at the time, and the rain smelled so good. With a condition such as congestive heart failure, you can't always get outside when you'd like to. When you're able, it's like a moment of freedom, and you want to enjoy every ounce of it.

My first challenge today was to wear ted hose [compression socks]. My diagnosis includes fluid retention in my legs. The ted hose should help. Talk about hitting home. I watched my dad wear these for many years. They are very binding and restrictive. After several hours, my legs feel heavier and itchy.

The next challenge I received said, "Your husband was afraid you were going to fall and asked the nurses to keep a close eye on you. You must sit at the nurses' station for 2 hours." People may think of that as an easy task. Not as easy as it seems. I am in a wheelchair, which is not comfortable. After a while, the pain begins to build in the lower back. Sitting in front of the nurses' station made me feel like I was in adult timeout! People walk by and stare. One person said, "You must not be behaving." Ouch! I had a very nice CNA sit with me for a while, and also another resident kept me company. I wasn't able to participate in any activities I had planned on. It felt like a punishment. There are other ways to keep an eye on someone without putting an invisible "dunce cap" or the label "in timeout" on the person. Sometimes, interaction is what a person needs—to be understood or heard.

My challenge for this evening was to get food on my clothes and once again go to the nurses' station and wait for someone to change me. I see residents spill things on themselves all the time. I allowed Bridgette to put tomatoes and cucumber salad (from my plate) all over me as though she had accidentally dumped my plate. I was anxious sitting at the nurses' station. People walked by and walked by again. I understand others need to be taken back to their rooms, but before taking another person, why not help the one sitting there? No one wants to sit with food all over him or her. Just as one CNA took a resident down the hall on her first trip, she politely came back to help me clean up. I was very thankful to get out of the messy clothes and into something clean.

### Jenny (Day 8)

Today, I was given some relief from the weights. After 8 days, I was in awe of how my legs felt without them. The less I had used my legs, the weaker they felt. I thought after wearing the weights, they would be stronger. I was wrong. After they had been removed for a while, I went to use the restroom. I only had to walk a few steps, but it felt so much farther. I see physical therapists walking with people every day. They go through challenges and struggles just to make it a few steps. I've watched residents come in without the strength to walk, get so much stronger, and go home. The courage and effort these people go through is truly amazing. They overcome their obstacle, climb the hill, and make it to the top.

I played several games today. I won a quarter at the horses and chocolate pudding at bingo. I haven't had a dime to my name since I moved in. When games have gone on while I was working, I would always ask "Did you win anything"? When you don't have anything and you win just a quarter, it's everything. It builds pride in the residents, a feeling of independence. Although small, they can call it theirs. The smallest things count. Whether a quarter, pudding, it doesn't matter—it is a big deal.

I've learned today that family life goes on without you. My husband came tonight for a short visit, and I expected to see my boys. They had other plans. It was a disappointment. It's difficult not to see your family all the time, not help in decisions, not know everything going on, and not take care of the home. You have to retrain yourself for a new life. Although hard to swallow, people you love still lead their lives. They come see you when they have time. You begin to feel guilty, even like a burden, when they could be doing something else even though you're happy to see them.

## "I still feel bad asking for help."

Bridgette has a chatty, beautiful personality. I stole the chatty part of her by not allowing her to verbally communicate, but I certainly could not take away her personality. It is what got her through the program. She persevered, using a communication board she carried with her to write on and convey her sense of humor.

## Bridgette (Day 2)

It's hard to joke around with people when you can't talk. When you finally get your point across, the moment has passed. Today in therapy, Liz challenged me to tie my shoe with one hand. It took a few tries, but I got it, and I was so proud of myself. A friend came today to keep me company, and that was nice. If having my family and friends come to visit means so much to me, it must mean so much more to the residents.

My shower yesterday wasn't that bad, but I couldn't have done it alone, so I appreciated the help. At first I was scared of being judged, but after we got started, I didn't worry anymore.

Today, I drew the challenge to lie in a wet bed. It was funny to see the reactions of those who were taking care of me, but for residents, I imagine it would be embarrassing. After a few minutes of sitting there, my clothes started to rub my skin raw, but I was determined to stick it out.

This morning, the call light in our room was jammed, so I took the risk of falling and transferred myself. I was nervous about it, and it actually took me two tries, but I got into my wheelchair and was able to communicate our dilemma to the maintenance man. People have teased me about not being able to talk, but it's actually not that bad. I slip up when people wake me up and I say "good morning," then I remember and cup my hand over my mouth and start laughing. It all works out.

I still feel bad asking for help because I don't want to trouble the staff, but they seem happy to help, and it's nice when they stop and talk for a few minutes.

## Bridgette (Day 4)

Today was interesting. I drew the challenge "You cannot make your needs known easily, and staff aren't taking the time to figure out what you want." The staff was supposed to not understand me even if they actually could. I guess being ignored isn't all that bad. I like to stay out of the way anyway. I tried to see if I could go to the bathroom before they put me to bed. To make myself perfectly clear on what I needed, I opened the bathroom door by the nurses' station and sat there until Nicole asked if I needed to use the bathroom. I thought it was funny, but, hey, they understood.

### Bridgette (Day 5)

I went to e-stim [electrical stimulation] therapy. Every time I did it, I laughed so hard because it felt funny and creepy. My mom couldn't be there to watch, so I asked Leslie if she could videotape it, not expecting an interview.

Needless to say, that did not go well because I couldn't keep a straight face the entire time. She asked me, "What's the hardest part of being here?" Still, I think it has to be the need to ask the staff for help.

Tonight, my challenge was to have my hands wrapped up to simulate contractures. I couldn't write. It was difficult, but I still didn't ask for much and the CNAs were patient enough to watch me point with a spoon. The big issue was when I had to go to the bathroom. The thought of my co-workers wiping for me made everyone involved feel uncomfortable. But with a little bit of imagination, we were able to slide a rubber glove onto my fisted hand and wrap that in some toilet paper and I managed.

This group lived in the nursing home for 10 days. The evening of July 3, 2013, the three of them decided that since they moved in together, they were moving out together. They were tired and wanted to be home with their families for the Fourth of July.

Every single day, residents are trying to prove to us and to themselves that they do not need to be in long-term care. Reading Chelsey, Jenny, and Bridgette's accounts of their experiences makes me think so much about this, how our residents try each day not to succumb to aging and dependence. I think we need to look at this even deeper.

Bridgette took the risk of falling by transferring herself from her bed to her wheelchair because her call light was jammed. Chelsey asked housekeeping if they needed help with anything so that she could feel useful and important again. Jenny recognized the challenges and struggles of residents who do not have the strength to walk, but also their courage and effort to overcome obstacles to "climb the hill, and make it to the top."

Most often, the first words out of our mouths are, "We are here to take care of you."

*We are here to take care of you.*

Sometimes I can imagine a sweet 93-year-old woman screaming back at us, "But I don't want to be taken care of!"

*We are here to take care of you.* That statement reinforces the fact that if a person can prove he or she can pick up the remote control from the floor, or get his or her own pants out of the closet, or, the big one, go to the bathroom without anyone's help, then he or she does not have to live in long-term care anymore.

Aren't residents really just trying to hold on to the pieces of who they are? And, if so, what are we giving them back in return? What meaning and purpose do they still have if they can't pick up their own remote control that they dropped?

Bridgette's story tells us about her fierce desire to hold on to the independence she moved in with. Whether we are 18 or 88, that desire does not really change. We still want control over our lives.

Do you sometimes see how the more staff or family members take from a resident the more in control that resident wants to be?

Stop making decisions about people without their involvement. Our residents should always be at the head of the table, in the driver's seat, and at the center of the conversation.

It was summertime when this group moved in. We are blessed with a beautiful patio that includes a garden, fountains, a gazebo, and a swing set for grandkids. It is a popular hangout on warm, summer days. Bridgette, Jenny, and Chelsey each found solace and made many new friends while spending time on the patio.

The one question from our elders that I hate most is, "Can I go outside?" It makes me feel embarrassed, for them as well as for myself. They must feel like a 4-year-old asking a mother's permission to go out and play. A woman who raised 13 children with little money or a man who fought in World War II should not have to feel the need to ask for my permission to go out the front door and sit on the porch for a while. I wonder how many people living in long-term care yearn to go outside but never ask. And how many people working in long-term care just assume elders have no desire to go outside because they do not ever ask? Think about Bridgette, who had to use a communication board, to make her needs known. It can be exhausting to go through so much effort to simply ask, "Can I go outside and get some fresh air?" How many elders just quit asking because it takes too much effort?

Encourage residents to go outside, feel the sunshine, listen to the stillness of the snowfall, and catch the raindrops on their tongue. As care partners, stop taking those experiences for granted and remember to encourage everyone living in your community to do the same. Our garden, fountains, and gazebo are for all to enjoy, but especially our residents.

# 9

How Long Does It Take to
Learn about Empathy?

> Alice: *How long is forever?*
> White Rabbit: *Sometimes, just one second.*
>
> —Lewis Carroll, *Alice in Wonderland*

AFTER A FEW YEARS, we began to ask ourselves how we could expand Through the Looking Glass to involve more staff. I recognized that not everyone was able to move into a nursing home for 3, 5, or even 10 days. I did feel, however, that everyone could sacrifice at least one whole day. So we decided to challenge those who had not volunteered to participate to move in for only 24 hours. It would not be mandatory. They would be paid for 8 hours, and the other 16 hours would be voluntary. An incentive to take part was a drawing to earn a free day off with pay during the month the person moved in.

This was enough incentive to encourage nine more staff members to move in to see what life might be like for a resident of long-term care. Each person then wrote a short essay about the experience.

Much like the previous participants, the essays shared a common theme that included loneliness and boredom, which continue to be the two biggest challenges we combat in long-term care. These were not new revelations for us. Although we were not at a point where we could suddenly make great improvements to fix these historical problems, we were able to invite nine more people to the table for conversations about the issues as well as possible solutions. This exercise opened up more minds and inspired more people to think. For those reasons, encouraging staff to stay for 24 hours served a great purpose in our culture change journey.

## How Long Is a Long Time to Live in Long-Term Care?

When we as staff talk about Through the Looking Glass, we are always amazed at how long some of the participants lived in the nursing home. With wide eyes we exclaim, "Kat lived there for eight days!" or "Can you believe they were all still there four days later?"

I remember interviewing Tayler when she decided to move out. I said, "You lived in the nursing home for four days. That's a long time." With a big sigh, she responded, "Four days is a *really* long time."

I think back to that conversation and feel like a hypocrite every time it plays through my mind. Four days is a long time? For whom is four days a long time? It is all a matter of perspective, is it not? I guess four days is a long time for a staff member who has moved in as part of an empathy exercise and who does not really have to be here. Is four days a long time for someone who moves into long-term care for short-term rehabilitation?

It is not a long time for the skilled therapists or the nurses or the staff working to take care of those in long-term care. They think, "I can't believe she was only here for four days." When we think of the consumers of long-term care, we think four days is a short time. What could be so bad about spending four days in a nursing home?

I posed the question "What is a long time to live in long-term care?" to a group of people I was presenting Through the Looking Glass to. Some said 5 years, 10 years, and even one week. Others said it depends on the person and why he or she needs to be in long-term care. One person said one day.

Perhaps it depends on the support you have from family and friends. All of the participants told me that the time went by faster for them when they were able to spend a lot of time with their families.

I asked Dorothy, who at the time had lived with us for more then 7 years, "You have lived here a long time—what has that been like for you?" Because of a debilitating bone disease, Dorothy had been dependent on others her entire life. She had learned to accept the life given to her and could always see the positive. She said,

> It doesn't feel like 7 years. It's gone by so fast. I'm not lonely here. I know some people are. I made the decision myself to come here. I cleaned out my own house and made the preparations on my own.

Another resident, Steve, shared with me that he wished he could go home, that there was "no concept of time here." He added,

> The calendar really screws with my head because to me all of the days just run together. I look at a calendar and I think, "How can that be? Where did the time go?" It freaks me out a little. When you are just sitting around in your wheelchair, it doesn't matter if it's Tuesday or if it's Saturday. You spend your time waiting for something, anything to happen. The loneliest part of the day is 5:00 in the evening when people are going home. It reminds me of my past life when I was working and I should be going home at 5:00, too.

Our days revolve around making choices for ourselves. We choose where we live, what kind of car we are going to drive, what we are going to eat, and who we are going to spend our time with.

For those living in long-term care, time passes very slowly when other people are making decisions for them.

How long is a long time to live in long-term care? That depends on who is directing the care. Staff-directed care takes away control from the person being cared for. Person-directed care helps to alleviate loneliness and boredom by allowing the person to control his or her own day.

# 10

# My 24-Hour Stay

*"So if we love someone, we should train in being able
to listen. By listening with calm and understanding,
we can ease the suffering of another person."*

—Thích Nhất Hạnh, Vietnamese Buddhist monk and peace activist

My own experience living as a resident in 2012 is one of the hardest challenges I have had as part of our culture change journey.

I was so nervous because, by this time, I thought our community had progressed by leaps and bounds, and I was feeling very optimistic about future changes. I was afraid I was going to see imperfections in our community that would derail my motivation to continue on the path of transformation.

I moved in on a Friday morning and went to my assigned room. It was so quiet and removed from my normal existence. I did not know what to do with myself. I was used to working there, not sitting around and listening to the day. My emotions were all over the place. I felt sad, lonely, happy, empty, content, angry, sympathetic, and empathetic. The hardest part of the day was the time of day when I usually headed home to my family. That day I did not, and I missed them.

During my 24-hour stay, I was told at least a dozen times, "I'll do that for you. Here, let me do that for you." At one point, when I was carrying my own dishes to the kitchen and a caregiver said that to me, I chided, "I want to do it myself. I have to feel like I still have purpose in this world." She probably thought I was cranky and needed a nap. If I had been an actual resident, maybe she would have spoken with her nurse supervisor about giving me an antidepressant because I was not adjusting well. Or perhaps she would have started a behavior-tracking sheet to document my "tearfulness" or "anger toward staff." I wondered if our residents even knew we are required by CMS to track their "behaviors."

As an administrator of a long-term care community, I know that there is a purpose for using behavior-tracking sheets. However, as a person just living life and reacting to certain situations, I cannot help but think it seems a little silly. It is perfectly normal for a person to feel a little sad about no longer being able to live without the help of others. I cannot stand the word *behaviors,* and I cannot stand the need for tracking them. It makes me feel as though we are not taking care of human beings, who are full of emotion all day long. We get angry with our spouses for forgetting to run an errand, or we become irritated with a co-worker for not doing something the way we think it should have been done. We cry because we had a stressful day. These are all very normal emotions. But add into the mix memory loss or a chronic condition related to getting older or not being able to bathe yourself and suddenly you are seen as having *behaviors.*

Behavior is a form of expression and a way of communicating unmet needs.

I am stepping on my soapbox here and asking everyone to please take that word out of your vocabulary. As human beings, we all react to the environment around us. Instead of tracking "behaviors," why not track "expressions of unmet needs" and use them as learning tools for better care partner support? Care partnering can be difficult with people living with memory loss or other challenges that affect their ability to communicate needs. I am not minimizing that. But there is still a *person* inside, and we need to *listen* to the whole person.

——— ◆ ———

About a year before my 24-hour stay, there was a man living in the nursing home whom I could talk to about anything. Bill was my "go to guy." Our conversations would always bring us laughter. One day, he and I were chatting about his neighbor who was dying, and Bill knew it. I kept trying to change the subject away from the obvious, but eventually Bill asked, "He isn't going to see tomorrow, is he?" I did not know what to say. It was an awkward moment for me. I answered, "No, Bill, he probably isn't." There, I said it. Silence.

In the previous few weeks, Bill had lost two neighbors, so this would be his third. "I'm worried I'm going to be next," he said to me. "What?!" I said, laughing uncomfortably. "Why would you think that? Do you think death is contagious?" He answered, "What if it is?"

*What if it is?* That conversation I had with Bill has stuck with me. I did a terrible job validating his feelings that day. I wanted to protect him. But he did not want to be protected. He wanted me to hear what he was really saying—that he was afraid of dying. Bill had been thinking about it. He was worried.

My 24 hours spent living as a resident provided me unique experiences, but one in particular made me think about that conversation I had with Bill a year earlier.

My neighbor, the man living in the room next to me, died the night I was living in the nursing home.

I heard his daughter begin to sob, and I knew what must have just happened. I lay there frozen for a minute. Being there as a resident, I did not know what I should do. It was a role I had never been in.

*Is death contagious?* In that moment, the question Bill had asked ran through my head. I could not help but wonder whether the other residents were feeling or thinking the same way as Bill had that day. I got out of my bed and went to console the man's daughter. I was the only "resident" who did. Not everyone was asleep yet. We had just said our goodnights a few minutes before. No one else came out. The place was silent with the exception of my neighbor's room.

Were people afraid? Or did they just feel helpless? I felt a little of both, as had Bill. It is difficult to know what to do or what to say. I made myself available, as a resident; not as an administrator. I offered to make phone calls. I met the priest at the front door, and I prayed. Doing all of these things made me feel less afraid, and they gave me a purpose. I was not just lying there wondering if I was going to be next.

That was how Bill had felt, but I did not take him seriously. I would from now on.

Bill passed away in the spring of 2014. When my phone rang that evening, I knew he was gone. I was heartbroken but so blessed at the same time. Bill had given me insight into my profession as a nursing home administrator that I had not had before. He was scared, and he taught me to be there for him. I needed to be there for him in that moment when I wanted to be selfish and make myself feel more at ease.

I think about my 24-hour stay often. Those hours spent on the other side of the door were powerful for me. They will always make me continue to strive for a better place for our parents and perhaps for myself when I need it and even for my children. That is the part that scares me the most about dying—that I am no longer around to ensure my kids care and safety. I need to know that I have done all I can for them, to have a place that loves them and holds their needs to the highest standard.

PART TWO

◦ ◆ ◦

# Lessons Learned

# 11

·◆·

# Changing the Way We Hire and Orient New Staff

## A Person-First Approach

WORKING IN LONG-TERM CARE is not for everyone. I am sure I am not the only person who has experienced the "Oh" reaction when you meet someone for the first time and are asked what you do for a living.

We receive applications from people who have never worked in a nursing home before. In fact, some have never even visited a nursing home. Of course, everyone in long-term care has had his or her first time working in the industry. As a result of our culture change journey, and also based on the experiences of those who have participated in Through the Looking Glass, I am much more particular about how we choose staff, especially the first timers, but also those on the opposite end, the ones who have worked in a lot of nursing homes.

Sure, you might be looking for a job, and, as with most long-term care communities, we might really need to hire CNAs or nurses, housekeepers, or cooks. But we want to hire someone who *wants* to work in long-term care. More specifically, we want someone who wants to work in *our* long-term care community. We are different. We are person first in our approach to care partnering with our residents. But we are also person first with our employees. This is a profession that is reciprocal in relationships. Our staff cares for our residents, but our residents also care about our staff. If as an employee you can allow that building of relationships to happen, it can be the most meaningful career you will ever have.

Like many other communities, we had experienced very high staff turnover. Turning that around was a primary focus of our culture change journey. Early on, Through the Looking Glass began to make a name for us and a lot of people were applying to work in our community. Our goal, however, was not just to have a bunch of people apply. We wanted the *right* people to apply.

When I talk about working in long-term care, I often say: "This isn't a fast food restaurant. Here people aren't waiting on you to make their double cheeseburger and fries. They are waiting on you because they NEED you." The residents need your help in fulfilling their basic needs, like going to the bathroom, eating, cleaning their clothes, or providing a clean place for them to live. But beyond the basics, we need people who will go even further to nurture, love, respect, and honor the elders who live in our community.

There is a really big difference between people who apply because they need a job and those who apply because they want to be here. We do not want people who just want to get paid for showing up. Show up AND be present. Being present is most important.

Working with the aging population is an honor. These are real human beings with great needs. They do not want someone taking care of them who they sense does not really want to be here in the first place. Guess what? Most people do not really want to have to live in long-term care either.

A few years ago, a resident came to me about a CNA who she felt had been rude to her when she asked if she could go out and have a cigarette. She said the CNA acted as though she did not have time for her. This had not been the first time I had heard this same type of complaint about this particular CNA. Right then and there, I decided to take a risk. I called the CNA into my office to discuss the concern the resident had raised. I started by asking, "Do you even *want* to work here?"

"Yes," she said. "I love my job."

I said, "Then show them you love your job."

The residents she was caring for did not think she even wanted to be there. They felt like a burden to her. She needed to prove to them how much she wanted to be there and how much she loved her job. I asked her to go home, pack a bag, and be back in an hour to be ready to live as a resident for 24 hours. I felt that if she did not want to give us that, then she should consider working somewhere else.

She left.

And then she came back with her overnight bag.

I was pleasantly surprised at her willingness to want to know how to do better.

I remember her coming to me the next day with tears in her eyes. "I am so sorry," she said. "I didn't know. I just didn't know." She learned personal stories about the people she had been taking care of. She became a care partner in those 24 hours. She was no longer that impatient caregiver.

She wrote me a letter about her stay:

> While staying at the nursing home, I learned that I needed to have a better understanding of how hard it is to be dependent on others. I need to remember no matter how frustrated I may get sometimes, the residents don't really want to be here and

that frustrates them more. I have also learned that during the evenings when there isn't as much going on, the time for them seems to drag on. Many of the residents talk about their family and how much they would love to be at home again. Staying here one night makes me miss home, too. Some of the residents think they can still do the things they used to before they got sick or hurt. It frustrates them so much when they realize they can't. For me to have patience helps the situation a lot, because when I rush the residents can tell, and it tends to make them uncomfortable and agitated.

This CNA invested herself in us, and she became like family. She grew and became a compassionate care partner. I was glad I took a risk that day, and she did as well. She could have easily said the heck with this place and found a job at another nursing home. Instead, she stayed, and we grew and improved together.

We need people who *want* to be here, working and caring about what they do and why they do it, as well as building relationships with residents to better understand their needs. If you are just out looking for a job, apply somewhere else.

That is a really hard stance to take when you really need staff. It is tempting to hire the person who did "pretty good" in the interview. You are thinking in the back of your mind how this person could be the answer to the hole you have on the midnight shift. "If I hire her now, she could be oriented and on her own by the weekend."

Do not do it.

Taking the stance to slow down the hiring process is an aspect of culture change that can create staff longevity in your community. I promise you.

## Hiring the Right People

So how do you hire the right people? First and foremost, stop hiring people on the spot. If you continue to hire the first warm body to walk through the door, you are only going to get a warm body working for you. You are not showing the person the value of your community. You are just showing him or her a place of employment. Because, really, there is a difference between a place of employment and a place where we are part of something bigger. Working in long-term care is not just a job, so please stop hiring people looking for jobs.

During an interview, I always ask the person what made him or her apply to work in our community. The answer I am *not* looking for is, "Well, my supervisor cut my hours and I need a full-time job." Or, "You are a 10-minute drive closer to my house."

The answers I *am* looking for are what the person knows about our community and why he or she applied to work here. Do they know we have a unique approach to caring for our residents? Do they understand what person-centered care really is?

When you are interviewing someone, spend a lot of time talking about your community. I always share that we are a person-first community and that if he or she works best with routine and in a task-oriented environment, then a position with us may not be suitable. The residents' needs come first. A scenario I often share is that when a person living in our community wants to go for a walk, we go along for the walk. If a resident wants to sit on the front patio, we join him or her. Most of the time the response I get is, "I can sit outside with the resident? I'm allowed to do that?"

"Not only are you allowed," I reply, "it's expected."

Tell the person about the progress your community has made in adopting a person-centered care approach and the community's goals for continuing to build on those successes. Make sure he or she knows your values and mission. Spend time introducing him or her to people who live and work in the community.

Also talk to the person about how your community is person first with employees and give examples of what that means. It is expected that everyone pitch in when a co-worker needs help. His or her job becomes your job because we are all working in the community for the same reasons.

Watch the interviewee's body language, but also pay attention to yours. If you are not excited and engaged in telling the person about the adventure he or she is about to embark on, then he or she probably is not going to be excited or engaged either.

I think of our hiring process like this: It is like getting something for free versus paying for it. You tend to value more the things you had to save for and earn versus things that were just given to you. Do not give away jobs for free. Make potential new hires earn a chance to be a part of your community.

## Staff Empowerment

Staff empowerment was a key goal of mine in setting up Through the Looking Glass. It was a hard goal to set, because I did not really know how to teach empowerment. And maybe it is something you cannot teach. But it is something that happened as a result of the program. I think when people see how far you are willing to go, the risks you are willing to take, and the values you hold to be true, empowerment becomes the culture of an organization.

As more staff participated in Through the Looking Glass, "Nothing about me without me" became a mantra of empowerment for the staff. Everyone became a leader in some way. This is still true today. The staff working at Aviston really are empowered to be decision makers. They know what the expectations are. Decisions are often made without me, and that is okay. Yes, I am the administrator of the nursing home, but that does not mean that I am the only one who can lead the "change." The administrator should be the guide. Discussions of change and decisions regarding care are made together with everyone's input.

## Consistent Assignments

In 2009, Aviston adopted the care practice of consistent assignments, which has improved the quality of life for both staff and residents. Working together as a group on a daily basis, staff are better able to anticipate the needs of residents and provide a deeper level of care through personal connections. Residents no longer have to re-explain or share their needs and preferences and are happier having relationships based on mutual trust and understanding with the same care partners each day. I can honestly say that our residents have been much happier and are comforted in knowing that their care partner knows them, as well as their family. Our culture change to person-centered care has given staff the ability to take ownership of the roles they play in care partnering with the residents. Staff satisfaction has increased and turnover has decreased.

I talk all the time about how consistent assignments have been a key factor in so many more positive transformations for us. For example, our considerable reduction in antipsychotic medications could not have happened without important staff involvement. In the last quarter of 2012, our antipsychotic drug use was 17%. By the last quarter of 2014, our use had decreased to 8%. Keeping antipsychotic drug use at a minimum could not continue to be possible without ongoing involvement with the people who know and partner with our residents everyday.

## Resident Hiring Committee

"Nothing about me without me" also became a mantra of empowerment for our residents. As part of our commitment to transform our care practices to a person-centered model, we decided that we should not be hiring staff without input from the people they would be care partnering with—the residents themselves. So in the fall of 2011, we created our first resident hiring committee, which consists of six to eight residents who interview applicants. The department leaders do the initial interview and reference checks, and then the top candidates are brought in for a second interview with the committee. The department leaders are not a part of the committee interview. It is a one-on-one conversation between the residents and the applicant. The decision to hire has to be unanimous among the committee members. If the committee says no, then we do not hire the candidate. We have to respect and honor their decision.

The committee members have a list of questions they ask of an applicant. These were adopted from another community that implemented this practice, Sunny Hill of Will County in Joliet, Illinois. Our committee modified the questions based on what they felt was important:

- Could you tell us what position you are applying for and what experience you have in this capacity?

- Do you know anyone who works here?

- What did you like or not like about your previous job?

- Describe your work ethic.

- Do you have the patience to listen to my requests?

- Are you willing to cross departments if they need help?

- If you are not sure what is expected of you, what would you do?

- Why do you want to work with elders?

- Describe to us what you know about resident-directed care.

- If you witnessed something inappropriate, what would you do?

- If I had a special request, how would you handle it? If you could not honor my request, how would you explain that?

- What will we talk about while you are caring for me?

- What else would you like to share about yourself?

Some people have asked me, "But do they ever really turn anyone down?"

Yes, they do, although it does not happen often. The process reveals what is important to the residents. I will never forget one instance in which an applicant came in for her interview in a very low-cut top. One of the elders said, "No, I don't want her. If she can't come in dressed appropriately for an interview, she won't dress appropriately for work, and I don't want to be looking at her boobs all day long."

When the committee has chosen to hire an applicant, the reasons have included that "she spoke directly to us," "she was very friendly," and "she seemed knowledgeable about the job." Because we are in a small community, the residents have also chosen someone because "she comes from a hard working family" or "her sister worked here and was a great worker." It is important to them that the person is confident and talkative. They are never very impressed when the applicant is quiet and they can hardly hear his or her responses.

Honesty is exactly what we are looking for from the residents when they share their impressions about an applicant.

The most important benefit of the process is that it gives the residents a voice in who will be there for them. It is their home. They are the ones who need the staff to be a part of their daily lives. Does it not make sense, then, that they are the ones to decide who will be a part of their daily lives?

We have taken it a step further and also made the committee part of a new hire's 30-day evaluation. The department supervisor goes back to that committee and asks them, "How do you think this person is doing? Is he or she meeting your expectations? What, if anything, do you think he or she needs to improve upon?" The department supervisor then shares that feedback with the employee as part of the 30-day evaluation.

## Elder Shadowing Program

By 2012, Through the Looking Glass had been so impactful in helping our staff see themselves as care partners that we wanted every single employee to participate. But how would we do this? We knew we could not make everyone move into the nursing home for two, four, or even eight days. We could, however, make it a requirement of our orientation process. And that is exactly what we did. We decided that all new staff must spend a day living as a resident before they can begin formal orientation to the position they were hired for. Called the Elder Shadowing Program, each new employee "shadows" a resident on each shift (day, evening, midnight), either consecutively within 24 hours or broken up across a three-day time frame. If a resident is in a wheelchair, then so is the new hire. If a resident chooses to stay in his or her room, then so does the new hire. And when the new hire spends the night, he or she has to sleep in a resident's room.

### Elder Shadowing Program

It is the policy of Aviston Countryside Manor that all new employees participate in the Elder Shadowing Program in order to gain a better understanding of what it is like to live in long-term care.

All new employees will be assigned an elder to shadow by their immediate supervisor. You must shadow an elder on each shift: days, evenings and midnights. This may be done in a consecutive 24 hours or broken up in a three-day time frame.

During your elder shadowing experience, you must "live" like the elder you have been assigned to. This means eating the same foods, attending the same activities, and experiencing the same level of dependency as the elder you will be shadowing.

After you have completed the program, please write a short paragraph about what you learned and how it will affect your relationship with those living in our long-term care community.

Not all of our department supervisors thought this was a great idea. I can remember sitting in our conference room with all of them and the looks on their faces when I shared my idea. Trust me. It was the complete opposite of elation.

There was a fear that no one would even apply to work in our community when they learned of the requirement. Those who were against the idea felt that "People aren't going to be able to commit to living here, especially overnight." My response: "If they aren't willing to give our residents 24 hours, why would you want them?"

Me against the world (or, in this case, about 10 people) was kind of terrifying. I knew my expectation was very high. What if they were right, and people just stopped applying? Then I guess they would be right. When you are trying to change the culture of your organization, not every idea is a great one. As a leader, you have to be willing to say, "If this doesn't work, we can find a different solution."

But I had been here before when I floated the idea of Through the Looking Glass. In this case, I knew our current practice of hiring people right away was obviously not working. I felt the risk (blank application forms collecting dust) was worth the benefit of hiring the right people to be care partners to our elders.

I pleaded, "Let's just take a risk. Do something no one else is doing. If it doesn't work, is it really going to be worse than our current practice?"

We had to do something different, which we did all eventually agree on that day in the conference room.

As with Through the Looking Glass, I called our professional liability insurance as well as the Illinois Department of Public Health about what we were proposing with the Elder Shadowing Program. Although my initial idea was to have new staff go through the program before we officially hired them, I was told they first had to go through the standard background check process. Okay, we could live with that.

Once we launched the program, some of our prospective new hires knew they could not go through with it. We had an applicant who learned about the shadowing program during his initial interview. "I don't think I can do that," he said. That is okay. We want sincerity. It eliminates having to devote staff time to orienting someone who is not really committed to who we are and what we stand for. Others needed support, understanding, and encouragement. I recall when a new CNA had completed her day and evening shift shadowing and all that was left was for her to spend the night. She called the assistant director of nursing from the parking lot. "I don't think I can do it," she said. "I just don't think I can spend the night in the nursing home." They talked through what she was afraid of—namely, not knowing what to expect. But she knew that if she did not spend the night, then she would not have fully completed her orientation process and could not work at Aviston. She did not follow through that night, but she did reschedule and was able to honor her obligation.

**Amanda wrote:**

I shadowed an elder from 7 a.m. until 6 a.m. the next day. My resident was in a wheelchair, so I was able to experience what it was like to be in a wheelchair for that amount of time. By the end of the day my back, legs, and arms were so sore. I don't think many people realize the elder's life of dependency until they actually "live" like the elder. I'm glad there are activities throughout the day, because it really made my resident's day. The Elder Shadowing Program really puts you in the elder's shoes. This was an eye-opening experience.

**Rachel wrote:**

I learned many things from shadowing a resident. For one, I learned how truly isolating living in a nursing home is. With a home filled with 80 or more people, it leaves little time for the staff to just sit and socialize with the residents. By the end of my day, I was yearning for any type of social interaction that I could get. I could not imagine being that isolated on a continual basis. I also learned how degrading it feels not being able to just get up and do simple tasks independently. It's frustrating to have to rely on someone for all your needs. Going forward, this experience has increased my desire to give the residents the best care possible. Even if it means making time just to socialize, or take someone to the restroom for the sixteenth time. It's their home. We are their family and my goal is to make living in their home a pleasant experience.

We had also tried the practice of having new hires live an 8-hour shift for three consecutive days to capture all three shifts. At the time, our workweeks were set up on an 8 and 80 system, meaning overtime occurred after 8 or 80 hours. We ultimately chose to go with a 40-hour workweek to allow new employees the option of either doing all three shifts in a consecutive 24 hours or spreading them out over three days.

I prefer to have new hires do the consecutive 24 hours. I feel that setup has a much more powerful impact. Our residents do not go home at the change of shifts. They do not get a break.

The Elder Shadowing Program validates a new hire's position. It creates the opportunity for immediate connections with residents as well as accountability. It makes it really hard to walk out after only a few days.

———— ◆ ————

Deep culture change transformation cannot occur if you have constant turnover in your staff.

Our Elder Shadowing Program, along with our resident hiring committee, decreased our employee turnover by 37% in the first year. That was huge for us, all of us—residents and staff. Think about what staff turnover does to the culture of your community. It drags it down. It is time-consuming and costly to interview and train again and again. The Elder Shadowing Program became a nonnegotiable for us. No matter what the circumstances, every new employee must participate. Many will argue that they do not have money in the budget to spend on a 24-hour resident shadowing program. Before you risk becoming stuck in that thinking, break it down. How much are you spending on job advertisements? How many extra hours has each department spent on orientation or re-orientation?

What I love about the resident hiring committee and Elder Shadowing Program is that the prospective employee is right away developing a bond with residents and vice versa. Give your residents a voice in who gets to work in their home, and new hires the opportunity to walk in the shoes of the people they will be care partnering with. How many of you have gone through the process of interviewing and hiring someone only to have that person not even show up for their first day? That happens less and less with these two practices. It is not easy to turn your back on people with whom you have already begun to connect.

# 12

• ◆ •

# It Only Takes One Candle
# to Light Another Candle

*"Just as one candle lights another and can light thousands of other candles, so one heart illuminates another heart and can illuminate thousands of other hearts."*

—Leo Tolstoy, *A Calendar of Wisdom*

FROM THE TIME Through the Looking Glass was first launched, and throughout our community's culture change journey, I have tried to get the word out about what has worked for us in adopting more person-centered care practices. When I came up with the idea for the program, it was to teach staff empathy in our community and put the focus more on understanding our residents' needs. I never imagined it would go beyond that. I did not foresee the attention the program would receive and the contagious effects it would have not only locally, but also state- and nationwide.

Since 2010, I have shared our story and successes primarily through conference and meeting presentations, although a few articles have also been written about the program. As a result, other communities have replicated or adapted Through the Looking Glass. Here are their stories.

•◆•

Monica Plymale, Assistant Administrator of River Bluff Nursing Home in Rockford, Illinois, facilitated the program in her community. The winner lived in the nursing home for 11 days. All of the participants were made to live as Medicaid recipients and had a monthly maintenance needs allowance of $30, an amount set forth by the federal government (and unchanged since 1972). As Monica explains, this was a challenge for everyone:

> All of our contestants were very vocal about how difficult that was, especially because their money was deposited into our bank, so they experienced restricted access, which made it that much more difficult. One of them wanted to go to the gift shop, but our bank was closed because it was on a Saturday, and she was worried if she spent that much money on a couple of items in the gift shop, she would be short later if she wanted something different. They all struggled with that, and I will tell you that one of the CNAs who participated wanted to start advocating to our state legislature about how difficult that was for a Medicaid resident.
>
> We did the contest only once in our home, but what an impact it truly had. From looking at how we treat our residents in their home to purchasing better equipment, such as better pillows. Who would have known how terrible our pillows were?

River Bluff edited raw video clips of their staff's experiences and use them annually as part of a training video for in-services on person-centered care as well as choice and dignity:

> Our staff enjoys watching it each time because it gives them a reminder of what they could be doing differently. We even caught on video an improper transfer with a Hoyer being

done on one of our contestants, so of course we use that as a learning opportunity.

While working for a company that designed long-term care settings, Jeff Ahl, an architect, decided to move into different care communities to see what living as a resident would be like from an architect's point of view. He expected to find countless problems with the physical environment in each home he moved into.

Jeff moved into seven homes around the country, from very traditional homes to multi-level communities in the middle of the city to new and modern settings. After hearing about Through the Looking Glass, Aviston Countryside Manor became the sixth community he lived in.

When Jeff embarked on this journey, the expectation that he was going to get the real experience of living as a dependent resident of long-term care made him really nervous. He found that in some communities he was made more dependent than in others.

Before moving into our community, Jeff and I talked about his expectations of being dependent. I also spoke with the staff who would provide personal care for him. They did not really know how to react to a stranger wanting to pretend to be a resident. It was a very different experience of Through the Looking Glass than what they had shared with their co-workers.

I also warned Jeff that the time frame of his scheduled move in was during our survey window with the Illinois Department of Public Health and that the chances of his stay and our annual survey overlapping were very high.

Well, guess what? Our surveyors did come that same week. But I was not at all nervous about Jeff being there. By this time the program had become very much a part of our culture. During the survey process, we did everything for Jeff that we would have done for a real resident. Jeff mentioned that, "One of the surveyors stopped by and talked with me for a little while. She said that she admired the fact that I was doing what I was doing."

When we have our annual survey, I always feel bad for the residents having to live with the added company and anxiety in their home. We always try to keep life moving along as normally as possible, but that can be hard when you are being pulled in a lot of different directions during the survey process.

I asked Jeff if having the surveyors in the community had affected his experience. He said that instead of living as a resident as he had intended, he became more of an observer by focusing more on the interactions between the residents and staff versus his own experience of being cared for. His perspective overall, though, was a positive one:

> In a nutshell, I learned that while I do have the ability to improve a resident's emotional state through quality design, the vast majority of issues I experienced were not a result of poor architectural design, but rather the result of a weak culture or poor relationships between staff and the residents or other staff members. Ultimately, the change in my approach to design of long-term care communities has been more about "how" I perform my work than it has been about "what" I design. My belief is that excellent communication should serve as one's minimum standard with a goal of achieving selfless understanding of the person you are communicating with. In all my research, I confirmed that every home is different. A successful home will be filled with residents and staff who know who they are and what they are about and who live in a way that supports the positive aspects of the culture each person brings to the home. It takes relentless and strong leadership to cultivate that culture and make sure it is in alignment with those who work and live there.

My experience has strengthened my resolve to advance change in senior housing. In fact, I believe we will never reach the goal of a perfect home for seniors because we are all different, and because culturally and socially we are changing all the time. So, I believe successful homes will be those that recognize they must always look to change to meet the needs and desires of those they currently serve with an eye on those they will soon serve. There are some amazing things happening in design and care in our industry, but in many ways we are behind the ball.

The name of the company Jeff co-founded, arCuretecture, was literally named as a result of what he had learned living as a resident in long-term care (Cu = culture, re = relationships).

Gary Glazner, founder of the Alzheimer's Poetry Project, became a resident of Aviston Countryside Manor for one week in 2013. He heard our Through the Looking Glass presentation at the 2011 National Pioneer Network Conference. Gary had attended the conference to talk about his innovative approach to using poetry to engage people with dementia. What caught his attention during our presentation was Chris, who was there presenting with me and who was one of our first participants in the program:

He went up to the podium, and you could tell he was nervous speaking in front of the huge crowd, but his was the most moving talk of the day. I thought to myself that if I ever have a chance to try something like he did, I would.

When Gary contacted me to participate, I recall that it took me a few days to even respond to him. I wondered why this world-renowned innovative thinker on creative arts engagement for people with memory loss from Brooklyn, New York, would want to stay in our little community. I was kind of star struck. Our small town has a population of just under 2,000 people. It was unbelievable to me that our program had caught his attention.

Gary's goal for moving in was to deepen the experience of his own work with elders by understanding what their lives are like. Through his work with the Alzheimer's Poetry Project, he is in control of what goes on, but when you move into a nursing home, you have to give up some of that control.

I talked to the staff and elders about Gary's request to move in. It needed to be a decision we all agreed upon. At first, I thought that maybe we would only let a few people in on who he was and what he was doing. I thought the secrecy of his purpose might help him get a fuller, more authentic experience. We decided against that idea because we valued the trust we had built with the staff and elders and did not want to jeopardize that.

Gary did move in and we had him share a room with Andy, one of our residents. We gave Gary a diagnosis that required him to use a wheelchair to get around. He also had paralysis of his left arm. Like our other contestants, Gary experienced challenges like urinary and bowel incontinence, drinking thickened liquids, wearing adult diapers, and eating puréed food.

Gary quickly fell into a routine. Breakfast, lunch, and supper—some days those were the highlights, as well as playing bingo every day.

Gary made a difference in the lives of our elders in the week he lived with us. One of his more profound experiences was with Mimi, which he details in his book, *Dementia Arts: Celebrating Creativity in Elder Care* (pp. 169–172):

Through my participation in Through the Looking Glass, I learned compassion, to slow down, what it feels like to slow down, and what being bored really feels like. And this brings me to the hardest moment of my stay at Aviston: saying goodbye to Mimi.

I met Mimi at breakfast my second or third day at Aviston. She was funny and quiet and recognized that, like her, I had my arm strapped down. Like her I was in a wheelchair, and like her I was in my mid-fifties.

I wheel over near her and ask if I can ask her a question. She says, "Sure." I take out my notebook and pen and get ready to write. I can tell she is curious about me carrying a notebook, so I tell her, "I am writing about staying here to help me get a sense of what it is like to live here. May I ask you, please, what it is like here?"

Mimi thinks for a moment and says, "It's boring here. That is what it is like, it is boring."

She then looks at me and says, "May I ask you a personal question?"

"Sure," I say.

She wants to know if I have had a stroke, and tells me that I have the same symptoms as she does.

"Have you had a stroke?"

"No," I say. I explain again that I am writing about staying here, and that Aviston has a program for people to stay and feel a little of what it is like to live here.

Mimi says, "And you are staying here for a week."

"Yes."

"And after your week is done, you are going to stand up and walk out of here."

Saying yes to Mimi, yes, I will walk away, yes, I am fine, yes, it is a learning experience, yes, I am free to leave, yes, you are here and cannot leave, and, yes, we do not say it, but, yes, you will die here or at a place like here—this is the hardest lesson in empathy that I learned during my time at Aviston and the hardest challenge I had faced, much harder than any of the other challenges.

"I think you're lucky," Mimi says.

Later, it comes back to me through the grapevine that Mimi has been telling people I am a spy. She says that I am always writing down notes, and the staff should be really careful what they say around me. People tell her I am here as part of a program, but she does not buy it and is sure I must be a spy.

I ask Leslie if she thinks it would be okay if I go back to Mimi's room, and she says she thinks it would be a good thing to do.

I wheel myself back there and Mimi looks up as I get to her doorway.

"May I come in and speak with you?" I ask.

"Yes," she says.

"I wanted to tell you thanks for writing the poem with me."

"Thank you," she says.

"I am always taking notes because I am trying to learn what it is like to live here. You have helped me learn that."

"You are not a spy?"

"No, I am not a spy."

"But I saw you talking to Leslie."

"Yes, Leslie is my friend and I do talk to her about my experience here."

"Did you tell her what I said about it being boring?"

"Yes, and Leslie wants to hear what you think. Is there anything you want me to tell Leslie for you?"

Mimi thinks for a while and says, "Yes, there should be more staff on this wing."

"Thank you, I will tell her. I have really enjoyed meeting you, Mimi."

"You are leaving now?"

"Yes."

"And you are going to get up and walk out of here?"

"Yes."

"You are so lucky."

Martin Bros. Distributing, a food service company to long-term care providers, also heard about Through the Looking Glass at a conference. They believe in the program so much that as part of their orientation process each new employee watches a DVD that documents Aviston's experience with the program. Gretchen Robinson, Marketing Dietitian for the company, explains why:

> We've used the DVD as a training tool to open the eyes of our sales team, who walk into long-term care communities. As sales reps, it's easy to focus on the people that you need to talk to and go on about your day; but it can't be "all about the sale."

One of our sales managers told me that after watching the video, he makes a point to greet residents sitting in entrances or walking down the hallways. He says that now he knows how much a smile and taking a few seconds out of his day can impact the well-being of a person. We have another sales manager who watches the video each year and ends up volunteering her time to serve in the community because it makes her aware of how much she is capable of giving back.

Jason Peterson, Territory Sales Manager for Martin Bros., feels that watching the video gives everyone a glance into their future and how they would like to be treated when they reach the point of losing most of their independence. "I talk to my sales reps about how not to think of people as 'beds' or 'per patient days,' but as your parents/grandparents," he said. Jason adds,

Depending on what capacity you deal with residents in a community like this, everyone can make a direct impact on someone's day. One of our main purposes is to help the community provide the best latter years living experience we possibly can. When you walk through the communities, don't just walk past these people, they have feelings and it doesn't take any longer to look them in the eye and address them with a smile or "hello/good morning." It should be everyone's nature to show the respect you expect. It has to be a very difficult thing to see people walking around or past you and wish you could still do those simple things that we all take for granted.

I really like Jason's statement, "It should be everyone's nature to show the respect you expect." It really is that simple. I remind people that when you walk into a long-term care community, you are walking into someone's home. We work where people live. Do we get that? Do we truly respect that? Are we reminding our vendors to respect that? We all work with contract vendors, whether it is food service representatives, skilled therapists, pharmacists, social service workers, or activity consultants. Do they all know what your community is about and what you expect of them as they work with your residents or your staff? Exceptions should not be made for them. Take the time to talk to them about how your community is person first and what that means.

Karen Sepich, Community Services Administrator at Bethany St. Joseph Corporation in Onalaska, Wisconsin, heard about Through the Looking Glass at the 2014 LeadingAge Wisconsin conference. After watching our DVD, she developed a plan to initiate sensitivity training in the eleven communities she works with, including assisted living, independent senior housing, and adult day care. All staff in each community participate in the training, which begins with watching the program DVD.

Karen has shared that after watching the DVD, many of their staff recognize that residents who move slower and take more time to process things, due to a physical, neurological, or cognitive impairment, need the staff to be patient and take more time with them. Another great outcome has been conversations about how they can encourage their residents to be empathetic with one another.

Everyone can use Through the Looking Glass in part or in whole. Whether you are an educator, architect, dementia specialist, or a vendor in long-term care, there is something for everyone to learn. Showing others the respect that you would expect in return should be a part of every care community's culture. Dignity, honor, and choice should always be in the forefront.

# Epilogue

## If You Want Culture Change, You Have to Take a Risk

*"I know who I was when I got up this morning, but I think
I must have been changed several times since then."*
—Lewis Carroll, *Alice's Adventures in Wonderland and
Through the Looking-Glass*

Do you ever feel as though you cannot make any real changes within your organization because your day is so full of chaos that you cannot actually get anything meaningful accomplished? We did, too. Sometimes, we still do.

Through the Looking Glass started out as a contest to teach empathy to staff as our organization started on a path to culture change, turned into a program to understand what person-centered care really is, and then just became a part of who we are as care partners. Eliminating personal body alarms, enhancing dietary choices, promoting continence, addressing residents' expressions of unmet needs, reducing the use of antipsychotic medications, putting into place consistent assignments, empowering staff and reducing staff turnover—the lessons we have learned and changes we have implemented have become embedded in us as well as our care practices.

One of the most important lessons we have learned along our journey is the significance of relationships. The Pioneer Network affirms this significance as part of their values and principles to bring about deep culture change: *"Relationship is the fundamental building block of a transformed culture."* This is so true. I will add that change cannot occur without trust, and that trust is built out of relationships. People are not going to be willing to take a risk, to take your word for it, if they do not trust what you are saying to be true.

If you want culture change, you have to take a risk. I know this probably sounds very cliché, but it is a lesson I have learned firsthand in guiding my organization to adopt person-centered care practices. Henry Ford once said, "If you always do what you've always done, you'll always get what you've always got." Some say that is the definition of crazy, and I often hear people in long-term care say that their job is driving them crazy. Then change something.

## Slow Down

Remember Nikki telling me she would slow down when I asked what she would be doing differently when she went back to work after participating in Through the Looking Glass?

Regardless of how busy you are, take the time to slow down. It will make a huge difference, and making a difference in one person's life *is* making a difference. Take the time to look for the missing sweater, eyeglasses, or the picture of the grandkids, because it is important. It shows that you care about and are aware of what is important to an elder at that moment.

One evening, I answered a call light for a woman who wanted her covers straightened up. She said she was cold and needed more blankets. As I was straightening and adding more covers, I let out a sigh. Immediately, I apologized. "That wasn't meant for you or about you. I'm so sorry." My thoughts had become distracted with something I knew my kids needed when I got home, and my frustration with that interrupted the moment I needed to be in. I decided to talk to her about it, not telling her the specific issue I was having with my kids, but instead talking about what it is like to be a mom and the joys and tribulations that go along with being a parent. She had memory loss and asked repeatedly if her daughter knew she was living here in our care community. I assured her that she did and that I had met her daughter and thought she was thoughtful and kind.

These conversations take time and patience. Forgive yourself when you mess up. Care partnering is hard work, but the rewards can be great.

## Stay Put

The temptation to quit and move on to a different long-term care community is great. Do not do it. If you are passionate about long-term care, stay put. How can any change happen if we are preaching to a different choir every few months? The same goes for owners. Give administrators a chance to make a difference. Lay out the mission and values of your community and educate and communicate together how your community can work simultaneously to grow and improve. I speak with staff from other communities who are disheartened and unfulfilled because they do not have consistent leadership.

Working in long-term care, it is hard to always have a positive attitude. We have so many misperceptions working against us. Television commercials from law firms that handle elder abuse cases, social media posts about nursing home abuses, and public perceptions are constant reminders of the negative connotations associated with the word *nursing home*. To make matters worse, some states do not financially support the industry in ways they should, so many communities struggle to meet the needs of their residents and staff.

These are not roadblocks, but instead hurdles that can be overcome along the path to transformational change. If you stay put. The hurdles make our jobs harder, but not impossible. If you stay put. The people living and working in long-term care need leaders who are not disheartened in the face of taking risks.

## Let the Residents Be the Leaders and the Staff Be the Followers

The residents are the leaders, and the staff are the followers. This may seem really small, but to the life of an elder it is really important. For example, during new staff orientations I am responsible for explaining our door alarm system. I do not like the fact that our doors have screeching alarms, but I do realize they are there for an important purpose. Here is what I tell new hires about the alarms: They are not to keep people in, but instead to alert us when we have missed a cue that someone wants to go outside. And when someone does go outside, we never redirect the person to go back inside. We follow along and join the person. It does not matter if it is raining, snowing, hot, or cold. A person who is 87-years-old and forgetful some or most of the time is not oblivious to the pouring rain or the quiet stillness of snowfall. Let the person be the one to experience being outside through his or her own senses. But go and be with the person. Be present with him or her in that moment. Not as a babysitter, but as a friend and care partner.

I had one of our Through the Looking Glass participants, Victoria, wear a WanderGuard® bracelet. I wanted her to know how it felt to be monitored at all times, that if she went outside the whole place would know. Remember how some of the participants did not want to use their call light because they did not want to bother anyone? Imagine how trapped inside Victoria must have felt not wanting to bother anyone by setting off an alert if she just felt the need to get some fresh air.

These scenarios may sound trivial, but they are a significant part of the culture of our care communities. Always put yourself in the other person's shoes in the moment. Instead of constantly redirecting, ask where the person would like to go, and follow along.

## Create Home

I remember a conversation I had with a resident after I had returned from a family vacation to Yellowstone. I was telling him how beautiful it was and asked if he had ever been there before. "I have been to Yellowstone," he said. "I have been all over the world. I was in the military and saw a lot of beautiful things."

I asked, "What was your favorite place?"

"Home," him replied.

I was suddenly at a loss for words. It was not an answer I was expecting. Home was what was important to him. Home was where his most cherished memories had been made, not traveling the world.

Home is where we feel comfort, safety, and security. Home is where we can build and share new relationships and memories. Traveling to great destinations creates wonderful memories, but home is where they are best preserved and shared with our family and friends.

You can create "home" where you are, but, again, it takes a willingness to stick it out.

## Change Something

I love the book *The Last Lecture* (2008), by Randy Pausch, who into the end stage of pancreatic cancer wrote about the life and moral lessons he wanted to leave his young children after his death. I loved it so much, I gave all of my department managers a copy for Christmas one year. It is packed with powerful advice. One piece of advice from Pausch that has stuck with me is, "Treat the disease, not the symptom."

Think about that statement when you look at some of the practices in your community. Constantly ask yourself if you are treating the problem or merely treating the symptom of the problem. This pertains to everything, from resident "behaviors" to always running out of jelly for breakfast. For those of you who are owners and budget people, you may already know that treating the problem costs a lot less money in the long run. It is treating symptoms that becomes very expensive.

It takes courage to treat the problem. It is easier to place bandages on the symptoms, but bandages fall off. They do not stick and neither will your constant efforts until you find the root cause of the problem.

Culture change takes a lot of work and effort. Like any major endeavor, it gets even messier and chaotic at the beginning, but then gradually over time you have organization and calm. Then that chaotic mess becomes worth it because you can stand back and feel really good because you know the change is going to stick.

Before we began Through the Looking Glass, I was the administrator who made decisions by putting out small fires every day. Now, I am a leader, or a guide, in our shared journey to transform our culture of care. We—myself, my team, and, most importantly, our residents—make decisions together. It was not an easy journey. There were a lot of risks involved. But you have to be willing to take a risk to make a change. You have to know and *trust* that everyone holds the same values as you do.

## Be There

*"We are here for the residents."*

This is a statement I hear in our community almost every day. I also hear it a lot when I am interviewing someone who really wants to work in our community.

*"Being here for these residents is what's important."*

That statement has a lot of depth to it. And I bet it has different meanings for different people.

Let me be clear: showing up for work is not "being there for these residents." It involves being present, being all in, and being in the moment, in all the moments that are important—and all moments are important. When you are hired to work in long-term care, you are making a commitment to be there for people who need you. You are committing to *being there.* So be there. They need you. If they did not need you, we would not have hired you. And do not let it be that sometimes you are committed and sometimes you are not. Be there and be committed in all moments.

I mentioned earlier how Through the Looking Glass helped us to become care partners with our residents. The definition of *partner* is a person with whom one shares a relationship. I think the key words here are *share* and *relationship.*

A new employee once said to me, "I'm not used to people sharing such personal relationships with everyone—residents, family, and staff."

That is what care partners are—people caring for each other, staff to resident and resident to staff. We become a family. We trust each other. We know we are going to be there for each other. If you do not have each other's backs, change is not going to work. If you continue to tear each other down by focusing on a person's weaknesses rather than supporting his or her strengths, a path straight to failure is your destination.

At Aviston we even became care partners with our surveyors. It can be done, folks. They are not the enemy. Take the risk, but involve *everyone* in the process.

In 2014, the team leader of our negative federal survey in 2004 recommended to another long-term care community spending some time with us at Aviston. She had seen how much we had grown, how Through the Looking Glass had forced us to see our care practices with a person-centered perspective. Our community had become a guide for what culture change transformation looks like, and the surveyor knew that. This was huge for us. The survey that stripped me down to the core of my professional existence built us up to become a community that could educate others. We would never have gotten to that point if we had not been willing to take risks.

Be willing to take a risk if you want culture change. Your whole community has to be built on trust for deep transformation to begin and ultimately be achieved. It is your community's deep imbedded culture, its mission and value, that defines who you are as a community and it is what will attract people to live and work there.

Be the person who stops leaving for the place that has better staffing, a bigger budget, or a more modern environment. Stay put.

Be the person who is committed to making a difference where you are. Be there.

Be the person who treats the problem, not the symptom. Things will change.

# Appendix

# How to Set Up
# Through the Looking Glass
# in Your Community

In thinking about how you want to use Through the Looking Glass in your community, consider the following tips and guidelines. Be sure to also review the FAQs section at the end of the book for more useful information.

———•◆•———

*Set expectations and goals for what you want to accomplish through the program.* Think about the pieces of empathy you really want to teach. For example, if you have a goal of eliminating the use of personal body alarms, have participating staff wear personal body alarms. First and foremost, however, look at your community's incident and accident data. Determine where and at what times most incidents and accidents occur that are setting off the body alarms and set up those same scenarios for your participants to experience. For example, make them wait to use the bathroom at the busiest times of the day, leave them disengaged at the dining room table, or hide their glasses. Also think about what transformations you want to achieve through the program. Maybe relationship building is something your community needs to improve. Or if you do not already use consistent assignments, ensure that each participant has a different caregiver for each shift and for each day of his or her stay.

*Decide what the rules of the program will be for staff in your community.* The rules we have used can be found in the Prologue. Adapt them to your own community. Write them down, post them, and hand them out to all staff.

*Include everyone in a conversation about the participants' expectations as well as those of the staff who will be responsible for caring for them.* Talk to all of the staff. I suggest small group learning circles in which everyone has a chance to speak and each staff member has the opportunity to ask a question or bring up a concern. This type of setting is less intimidating and gives everyone in the room an equal voice. Co-workers will want to know what are the expectations of them. Will they be helping their peers with going to the bathroom, bathing, and getting dressed? As our program went on, the level of comfort improved for those caring for the participants. With the first group, I was not sure how far I wanted to push the comfort level. I was afraid people would not participate if I pushed too far. As we went on, the yearning to know more about the needs and challenges of the residents grew and so did the level of understanding of the people taking care of the participants.

*Meet with your resident council and include their family members in the conversation as well.* These are the most important people to ask what they would like to see happen as a result of the program. Ask your residents who would like to volunteer to have a program participant be their roommate and talk about what that would mean. Let family members know about the new roommate as well. We approached the roommate situation similar to how we would with any new person moving into our community. Anytime a resident is getting a roommate we always discuss this with the resident and/or a family member to get their approval.

*Let your state surveyors and your insurance company know what your community is trying to accomplish through the program.* It may be to reduce staff turnover, reduce falls, improve resident engagement, and so forth. It is always a good idea to be proactive in informing these entities because they may think of an issue that you did not. We have never had a problem with surveyors or our insurance. Both entities were fully supportive of our program.

*Find out how many staff want to participate and pick a move-in date.* Based on how many openings you have, decide if you are going to let everyone move in at once or just one or two people at a time. With our first group, they moved in when it worked with their schedules as opposed to all at the same time. This had advantages as well as disadvantages. It worked better for the staff who had to care partner with the participants because it was not a large influx of new "residents." One disadvantage was that the last person to move in knew how long she had to stay to win the grand prize. Another disadvantage to people moving in individually is that they did not have the group support that was felt when participants moved in together. This could also be viewed as an advantage in that you may want a participant to feel the loneliness of the situation. Discuss the advantages and disadvantages with your community and decide what will work best.

*Make up diagnoses.* They do not all have to be a diagnosis that makes a person completely dependent. Mix it up. You can always make an independent person's diagnosis harder the longer he or she stays, such as dealing with the effects of a fall or hip fracture or infection. Above all, base your diagnoses around what you are trying to achieve through the program. One suggestion is to select a care plan of someone already living in your community and have a participant live by that care plan.

The following are some sample diagnoses you can use and how to simulate them:

- *You are legally blind.* To simulate your blindness, you must wear vision-impaired goggles at all times. You depend on staff to take you where you want to go. You were released from the hospital with a diagnosis of *C. difficile.* You are incontinent of bowel and wear disposable underwear at all times.

- *You have end-stage cardiac disease.* You have decided to have hospice care. You are not able to get out of bed due to excessive weakness. You are unable to get up to use the bathroom and cannot tolerate sitting in the dining room for meals. You must use a bedpan and eat your meals in bed.

- *You have a fractured right ankle.* You will need to wear a supportive boot and cannot bear weight on your right foot. You will need to have a leg rest on your wheelchair to support your right foot. You will need to use a bedside commode until you can be evaluated and cleared to go to the bathroom by yourself.

- *You had a stroke and are moving into the nursing home because you are no longer able to take care of yourself.* Your stroke occurred on the right side of your brain, so you are weak on the left side of your body. You will wear a 3-pound weight on your left arm and a 5-pound weight on your left leg to simulate the weakness caused by the stroke. You also have weakness in your tongue and muscles of your face and will be on a puréed diet with thickened liquids. You are unable to transfer yourself or walk. You have orders from your doctor for physical, occupational, and speech therapy.

- *You have a right hip fracture and are confined to a wheelchair.* You cannot bear weight along your right-lower extremity. You are experiencing confusion from time to time and try to get out of your wheelchair without assistance. You must be kept in a supervised area when in your wheelchair or not in bed. You are not to be left unattended in the bathroom or during bathing.

*Involve a staff participant's family.* Sometimes family dynamics are a challenge when care partnering with our residents, so including a participant's family as much as possible can enhance the experience of the program. Include them in completing the admission paperwork and moving in personal items, and call them when something comes up that they need to be informed of. Some families visit often and others hardly at all. Some families say they are coming to visit and never show up. Both of these scenarios happened with our groups and they had an effect on the participants that was not expected. Some felt increased loneliness and less control (because their family would make decisions for them), while others felt more supported because their family would visit often.

*Move-in day!* What does the move-in process look like in your community? Do your best to replicate that process for the participants. Also talk to them about why they want to participate in the program and what they hope to accomplish, both personally and professionally. Some answers may surprise you. Remember Nikki, who said she moved in because she needed to remember why she was still working in long-term care? If she did not find that answer while living as a resident, she was going to change careers. Knowing the reasons for moving in also helped guide me in deciding what challenges they should experience. Also ask the participants what they are least looking forward to. This will also give you some ideas for the challenges you will give the them.

*Decide how you want to set up the challenges.* Set up challenges that are thought provoking and that force participants to think about what they may be taking for granted with respect to a resident's experience of long-term care. We have chosen challenges that our elders face every day, from losing a pair of glasses or an item of clothing to dealing with incontinence, having no visitors, or treating a pressure sore. We also set up challenges based on a declining diagnosis (e.g., worsening chronic heart failure or a fractured hip caused by a fall due to worsening Parkinson's or dementia). Beyond challenges that focus on physical losses, be sure to also focus on mental and psychosocial losses, which are what will be the catalyst for deep systems change within your organization. Challenges as simple as losing someone's glasses, not allowing a person to brush his or her teeth daily, or having a person wear a bracelet that alerts staff when he or she goes outside can give someone the sense that he or she no longer has control over his or her daily life.

*Ask the participants to write down how they are feeling every day.* Have participants keep a daily journal of their experience or have them blog about it. Capturing everything they take part in and how they feel day-by-day is a crucial part of the program. Post journal entries online or have the participants share them on a blog. It is important for other staff to read about the participants' experiences of the program.

*Have cameras ready!* Record video of the participants every day, several times a day. You can use the video recorder on a smartphone or tablet to capture each participant's experience of the challenges they are given. As with journaling and blogging, this is a great learning tool for other staff members and a great way to look back and see what was accomplished. Take a lot of pictures as well. Pictures are worth a thousand words and can be eye-opening in showing a participant his or her physical and emotional decline.

*Ask a lot of questions of the participants, the elders, and the families while the program is going on.* These questions will be the key to change in achieving the goals you want to accomplish through the program. Get as much feedback as possible. Encourage the participants to think about how they would apply what they have learned through their experience when they go back to being care partners. Ask family members what they wish the participants knew. Most of us have no idea how it feels to be a family member of someone living in long-term care. Last but certainly not least, listen to your residents. What are they saying to you? What would make a difference in their daily lives if the participants really knew how it felt to be in their shoes? Remember, this is a learning tool for everyone!

# Frequently Asked Questions

*Did you have to get approval from the Department of Public Health to do the program?*

We did not get any kind of formal approval to do this program. I contacted our attorney and the Illinois Department of Public Health and let them know what we were going to do. They could not think of any reason why we should not do the program.

*Do the participants sign waivers?*

We did not have the participants sign a waiver. The participants were made aware of the rules of the program and agreed to them.

*Have you ever been worried one of the participants would develop a pressure sore?*

No participant has ever developed a pressure sore or been hurt during their stay with us. Remember, these are generally very healthy people who are moving in with us.

*How does the staff feel about taking care of someone who is not really a resident?*

This was one of the hardest challenges the first time we did Through the Looking Glass. Everyone is busy, and it was frustrating to the staff at first to have to take time to care for someone who did not really need care. This gradually became less of an issue as the years of doing the program progressed. They want to provide a learning experience for the participant as well as for themselves as care partners. And the staff, of course, are going to choose to take care of a real resident before a pretend one.

*Did you find it was easier to manage the staff's experience of the program if you had one participant at a time move in versus several staff members moving in together?*

Yes, I did find it easier. When I had five participants all living there at the same time it was really busy because it was doing five challenges at a time, interviewing and filming, and so forth. Having only two people participate at a time would be a lot more manageable and having just one person would be even easier. The less people who move in at one time is also easier on the staff caring for them.

*Do the participants get paid for being in the program?*

Yes and no. They get paid for the time they would have normally been working. All of their other time is their donation to learning what it is like to live as a resident in long-term care.

*Do you do Through the Looking Glass only for nursing staff?*

No, all types of staff have chosen to participate in the program: RNs, LPNs, and CNAs; DONs; housekeeping and laundry staff; OTs and PTs; activity and social services staff; and dietary staff. Anyone employed by your organization can benefit.

*Has anyone ever resigned while participating in Through the Looking Glass?*

No one has ever resigned from their position in the community while participating in the program.

*How have the elders felt about being a roommate for a participant in the program?*

We always ask permission from an elder before he or she is paired with a participant. The elders have for the most part enjoyed and been fully supportive of what their care partners are learning. They like the company, and they like telling them about life in long-term care and what their life was like before they moved into the nursing home.

*How did the program change you all?*

It changed the way we look at our care practices and approach issues. It opened our hearts and minds to change. We often now think first about what is most comfortable for a resident rather than a task that needs to be done.

*Has anyone ever moved into the nursing home secretly posing as a resident to assess the community's approach to care?*

No, however, many people have asked us this question. I have even had ombudsmen from different areas say they should secretly move into nursing homes in their own regions. We have never considered doing any part of the program "undercover." Relationships are built on trust, and relationships and trust are really, really important to us. Communication and teamwork are also important, and we think we can tackle challenges with all of those building blocks (relationships, trust, communication, teamwork).

***What life lessons have you as an administrator learned through this program?***

I have learned a lot about trust and communication. All of our jobs are hard in long-term care. There is not one job that is not emotionally stressful at times. Every piece has meaning and every piece is needed. I say this because it is so easy to get caught up in the hustle and bustle of the day. We all know that some days can be chaotic and there is a desire to want to close our eyes to the needs that are causing the chaos. I have learned to be a better listener. Listening takes a lot of practice. As an administrator, we want to fix things; but sometimes listening is fixing. So, I think the three life lessons I have learned from this program are *trust, communicate,* and *listen.*

***If I am an administrator and want to pitch Through the Looking Glass to my corporate office, summarize what you would tell them to persuade them to agree to it. Include what I could change to make up the money I would spend doing the program.***

This is the hardest question to answer. It comes up at every presentation I do. "I would love to do this, but how much does it cost?" or "My corporate people won't let us do this." My suggestion would be to take a look at the amount of money you are spending on staff re-education. Not only the cost of staff re-education, but also the time staff are clocked in to be re-educated. Look deeply into the in-service plan you already have and ask yourself what is working and, more important, what is not working. Determine how much money you are spending in the not-working-so-great-for-us column. How does it compare? Take a look at the money you are spending on recruiting and orienting new staff. Also take a deep look at staff retention. And then ask yourself, based on our own experience, whether implementing Through the Looking Glass, or even an Elder Shadowing Program, might actually save you money.

*If the corporate decision makers do not approve the program, what would you suggest I do instead to incorporate more change in my facility.*

Again, look at what you need to change. Then look at why it is a problem. Do a root cause analysis, or, as I like to say, treat the problem, not the symptom. Involve everyone in the discussion and get everyone excited about the possibility of deep change. Change is scary and fun and exciting and terrifying all at once. Acknowledge that. It is okay to let everyone know you are scared, too. The end result will be worth it.